Be **Free,**
Be **Slim**

7 Keys
to Total Victory
Over Food and
Your Body

Martine Wilkie

www.BeFreeBeSlim.com

BE FREE, BE SLIM
Copyright © 2010 - Martine Wilkie

English translation by: Sylvie Habel, Claude Liboiron and Marlène Bilodeau

Revised by: Marlène Bilodeau and Fernande Tremblay

Cover and layout: Betty Gurvits

Original French Title: "Sois libre, sois mince par la Parole de Dieu"
© 2008, Éditions A&M.

Published By:
A&M Publishers
600, rue Pierre-Caisse, C.P. 40013
St-Jean-sur-Richelieu,QC, Canada, J3A 1L0
www.AllenMartine.tv
ministries@wilkieministries.com

All biblical quotations are from the *King James* version of the Bible.
Bold characters in the biblical quotations are added by the author.

ISBN:13:978-1502422057

Legal deposit – National Library and Archives of Quebec, 2010
Legal deposit – Library and Archives Canada, 2010

Printed in Canada.

Dedication

This book is dedicated to My Lord and Saviour Jesus Christ, who saved, delivered, healed and restored me supernaturally. I am now free and I feel good in my body. You have erased so many years of hurt and suffering by your powerful hand. My life gives you all the glory. I glorify your name each time someone compliments me, because I know that it is You who delivered me from this burden. I also know that You want to do the same in the lives of others. Words are not strong enough to express the gratitude and the love I have for You. My life now expresses it to You in a powerful way through my passion for serving You full time and spreading the Good News of the Kingdom of God. Thank you Lord! May this book powerfully touch and transform lives for your glory, because You are alive and remain the same yesterday, today and forever. To You belongs all the honour and the glory!

Acknowledgments

To the love of my life, Allen:

I am so grateful for everything you have done for me. Your love, your encouragements, your constant support, your prayers and all the words of life you spoke over me literally transformed my life and my body. You met me when food and my body tormented me. By your obedience to the Lord and seeing me with the eyes of your heart, I am today a happy woman, free, fulfilled, and accomplishing myself day after day. You spoke words of love and life that strengthened my soul and I am the woman I am today in great part because of you. You uplift me, you love me and I am so blessed to be your wife. Thank you for being at my side. Together, we fight the good fight and go from glory to glory. You are an exemplary man of God, and I thank you again for having been and continuing to be a man of integrity in my life with the Kingdom of God mentality! May God fulfill you beyond your wildest thoughts.

I love you!
Martine

Special thanks to:

Eric Beaulieu, Chantal Frégeau, Véronique Charpentier, Betty Gurvits & Caroline Leclerc.

The completion of this book was made possible in great part by your generous donations, expertise, professionalism, and all the time you invested. May God greatly bless you!

With Love In Jesus
Martine

Table of Contents

Section Three: The 777 Program -
The 7 keys for absolute victory in 7 minutes a day for 7 weeks

Foreword

Michel Gagnon's Testimony

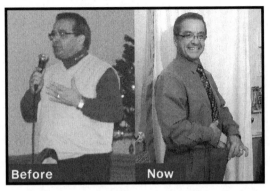

Before   Now

*M*y wife asked me to attend the "Be Free, Be Slim" course. I was reluctant at first, because I thought that course was designed exclusively for women, but I finally obeyed to my wife and we both registered to it.

I was a bit shy in the beginning because few men were attending, but my intention was mainly to observe and listen. Towards the end, I really decided to follow the teachings and I was motivated to fully get involved. I was convinced it would benefit me for multiple reasons.

Throughout my childhood, my mother expressed her love and affection by serving us all kinds of treats and desserts... This was part of our family traditions. Seldom was a meal served without dessert at the end. As time went by, this type of treat became for me a source of satisfaction. But I came to realize that the benefits were not that great for my body.

The teachings of Pastor Martine, transmitted with great intensity, have awakened in me the desire to get totally involved and to apply the principles of the "Be Free, Be Slim" course. Every week, we received a CD containing a daily coaching to listen to and I put at work the teachings received in the morning. From that moment on I saw the power of God's Word, but especially the effect of the power of the Word upon my body, thus, the importance of decreeing and proclaiming God's word over the latter. Unfortunately, when we go through difficulties like rejection, lack of love, loneliness, we have a tendency to compensate with something else that fulfills us. Personally, I found loophole in food. I had tried many diets, different types of weight loss programs, and of course I lost weight, but after a while, I regained it nearly in double.

What I liked about this course was that dieting and weighing were out of question. We could and still can eat what we desire when we are hungry: "If you're not hungry, you don't eat, but when you're hungry, you eat and stop when you're full." During the course "Be Free, Be Slim" I also kept hold of a very important key among the seven ones that were teached and it concerns the one that teaches us to compensate our need to eat by the desire to nourish ourselves with the Word of God.

I truly listened to my body, and realized that I was not eating three meals a day anymore. Sometimes we think we are hungry, but in reality, our body shows us that we may just need water. So I began to drink a lot of it. I discovered that by picking up this habit and decreeing words of life on my body, I started to really lose weight. I couldn't believe it! Yes, it works! The Word of God says that if you believe, you receive. We have received this power from the Word, and with the course I started to decree victory out loud over my body.

I took hold of the principle that we have the authority to speak to our soul and our body. I started experimenting special things like silencing the spirit of gluttony when I walked past a bakery that emanated enticing smells. I began to take authority over the negative tendencies I was entertaining in my life, such as buying two bars of chocolate every time I walked into a convenience store. I allowed myself to be tempted... It was the enemy who was toying with me. One day I said: "No, it's over! You no longer have a hold on me, spirit of gluttony!" Reading the Word of God, I realized that I had the sin of gluttony... I ate, I ate and ate! I had been alone for almost twenty years and had found comfort in food. Yet, I was not feeling well.

I really understood through the "Be Free, Be Slim" course that we have the authority to say no to the spirit of gluttony that comes against us, for the well being of our body. I really started to proclaim and command to my system to function normally using the divine authority I received. I began to talk to my liver, to my body... It has been dramatically transformed. My weight loss is visible to all who knew me from before. What is wonderful is that people around me can also see changes other than the weight loss. Hallelujah and glory to God!

In the course, Pastor Martine also teaches us about fasting, praying, sowing seeds and by applying them, I saw the difference. This had a major impact on my body. I started to fast with disconcerting ease. I told myself: "My God, I'm not hungry. It's easy to fast!" I also spoke to my body, **"Body, you**

are supernaturally restored in the name of Jesus Christ!" I realized that I ate half of my plate and that halfway through the meal the Holy Spirit showed me that I was not really hungry. I would have never left half of a steak on my plate before! I started to eat less because in the end, I felt that I did not really need to."

A year and a half ago, I weighed 220 pounds (100 kg), of which I lost almost 55 pounds (25 kg) after a period of one year. I went from a waistline of 40 to 36. I made people happy around me by giving away my old clothes. I work in the automotive field, and I am in contact with the public. Everyone, who knows me, tells me about my weight loss.

This is a course I recommend to everyone because it was a total success for me. It has not simply been a physical success; I also felt the benefits at spiritual and emotional levels. Today, I am truly convinced in my heart that it is not over... This is another way of life, another language, and a different lifestyle with my wife. I recommend it to all couples! Conversations with my spouse are more edifying because we encourage each other. We are a couple renewed by the power of our words. My wife has also lost considerable weight through these teachings. Moreover, she gives her testimony at the end of this book. In closing, I urge you to take this course and decide to take advantage of this teachings; then you will obtain an absolute and fantastic victory! **The Word of God is powerful!**

Michel Gagnon
Brossard, Quebec, Canada

Introduction

I would have so enjoyed reading a book like this one a few years ago! A book that could provide me with a lasting solution to a problem I wanted to eliminate in my life forever... a problem that weighed heavily in the balance, not only physically but also emotionally and psychologically. I read so many books on the subject! Several of them give advice on how to eat well and lose weight, but none could deliver me of the mental obsession I was constantly facing regarding food and my body.

All I wanted was to live the life of someone who had always been free and slim with his way of eating. I lived a real nightmare by imposing dietary restrictions on myself that you could not think of. I could not bear it anymore! I wanted to get out of this deadlock, but did not know how. I did not want to live my life with restrictions forever.

My desire was fulfilled! I am living proof of God's work, and this book is its testimony. I am really happy to bring you the revelations that my husband Allen and I have received from the Lord in the course of several months. Today, I live the life of a person completely free with food and perfectly well in her body.

I firmly believe that we have not received these revelations only for ourselves but for you also. I did not want to be blessed and go back to my life alone in my corner and keeping silent about this miracle. Through the encouragements of my husband, God put in my heart to share with others what I had received. After all, that is what the Kingdom of God is all about. It is about others. If you take advantage of these revelations, you will be blessed, delivered, and feel well in your body.

I knew for a long time that one day I would write in the purpose of being a source of blessings for others. However, I would have never believed or thought that my first book would be about alimentary and slenderness. God is so great and powerful! He sees the needs of His children and one of these major needs is physical and mental health. As the writing project moved forward, I was astonished to see how vast of a social phenomenon eating disorders and obesity really was throughout the globe. I am convinced this book will bring a revolution by helping God's people to walk in physical and emotional prosperity.

Will This Book Bring You a Solution?

Perhaps you've already read several books on weight loss, and you wonder if this book will offer a real solution to your problem. Perhaps you wonder if it's possible to end this problem once and for all in your life. Maybe you've tried several methods to break free: An operation, therapies, medical treatment, several diets, hypnosis, "miracle products", exercises, etc. Having tried all kinds of possible and impossible diets myself, after three years of therapy and exercising excessively to lose weight and having used various "miracle products", I can assure you that all these methods failed because I had not targeted the true root of the problem.

Two Specific Objectives

By writing this book, I have two objectives in mind: First, I want to be a source of inspiration for you since I have been completely delivered from this struggle in my own life. My second objective is to channel the seven keys that have brought a complete victory in my life, and to share them with you. You will be amazed to see how quickly you will get durable results in your life. I want you to look at yourself in the mirror with satisfaction and be proud of yourself, happy and having pleasure with food. These 7 keys will allow you to feel great in all occasions. No more diets! This book is based on the best principles that will allow you to live a free life, without deprivation, and in slenderness through the power and the truth of the Word of God that transforms you spiritually, mentally, and physically. Glory to God!

The powerful teachings you will find in this book are not presently taught and brought to light among God's people. Yet, each of us knows someone who is struggling with one or many of these problems. This book covers various topics related to food: deprivation, obsession, repetition diets, guilt, eating disorders, overeating, etc. You will certainly recognize yourself in the profiles presented in the book. Having gone through these battles myself, I can tell you that no one deserves to live through them.

Now, the time has come for you to establish new habits, change your perception and your behavior around food and especially, eliminate your bad programming. You will go from victory to victory, success after success if you persevere.

Do not lose sight of your goal! Be vigilant! Take charge of your life as I did myself, with the support and prayers of my husband. Take the road to success by reading and re-reading this book. Get diligently nourished through the revelations and principles and you will win a great battle... It all starts with one small step, then another... It is by knowing the multiple advices, the statistics, the information, the exercises, the secrets, the prayers, and the seven important keys that fashion the 777 Program that you will reach your goals of freedom and slenderness!

The 777 Program

The 777 Program consists of seven keys that you will follow for 7 minutes a day during 7 weeks on a consistent basis, day after day, week after week. **Follow this program and repeat it until you reach your personal goals.** Please refer to Appendix 4 for the application grids of the 777 Program you can use to help you manage the achievement of your goals. It is of the utmost importance that you remain consistent! Falling is not that serious; not getting up is!

These 7 keys are not only for seven weeks, but they will accompany you the rest of your life. It takes about 21 days for a human being to develop new habits. Through this program, you will establish a new awareness and a different attitude toward food and your body and it will forever bring a revolution in your life!

This Book is For You

This book was written for you, so you can get your victory. I am absolutely convinced that if you keep this book within sight during the next 7 weeks, if you read and re-read it every day of the week, you will experience a complete victory in your life! You will be a subject of glory for our God! Do not skip any steps! The first two sections of the book are as important as the third one, which contains the 7 weeks 777 Program.

Many of you will discover these principles for the first time, while others have heard of them in one form or another. You will find these principles presented under a new angle that will help you understand them at another level. My goal is to see you apply this knowledge in your own life. It is time to free yourself once and for all from this battle with food and your body by the Truth of God.

These 7 keys are not only for 7 weeks, but they will accompany you the rest of your life.

Go! Charge! Meditate! Apply! Persevere!

And You Will Be Victorious!

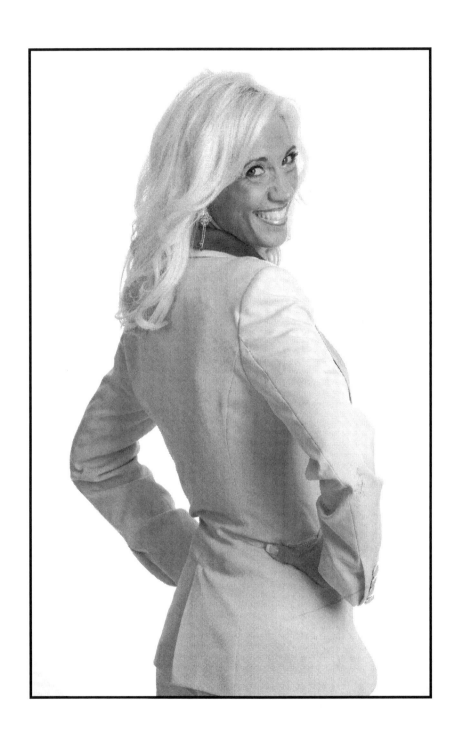

Section One

EATING DISORDERS AND OBESITY: A GLOBAL SPIRITUAL PROBLEM

"For we wrestle not against flesh and blood, but against principalities, against powers, against the rulers of the darkness of this world, against spiritual wickedness in high places."

Ephesians 6:12

1. A LITTLE ABOUT ME... AND YOU

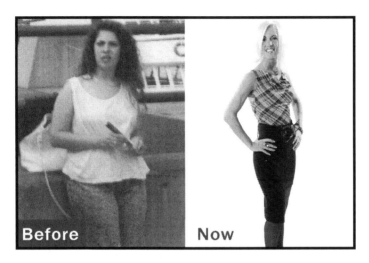

Before   Now

My Birth and My Family Legacy

*I*t all started when I was conceived. Yes! When I was conceived! I was born in a family where weight issues and perpetual dieting constantly affected all the women on my mother's side. Weighing only 6 pounds 6 ounces at birth, I clearly had no apparent weight problem... Growing up, I saw my mother lose and regain weight. She tried all sorts of diets and would constantly talk of her attempts to get a thinner waist and feel good about herself. I grew up with aunts and cousins who faced the same situation as my mother.

When I was 5 or 6 years old, I was fairly slim and was never concerned with this aspect of my life. I was doing gymnastics and swimming, and felt good physically. During that time, my older brother felt his mission in life was to pester me. I believe that one of his favorite pastimes was to anger me and make me cry **as it happens in so many other families**. One point on which he had the most success with was to call me "wonder fatso". He had even turned it into a song! My soul, without knowing it, recorded these words spoken over me and I hated hearing that song!

Self-Esteem

Whenever he sang these words to me, I started to cry and I would isolate myself. As far as he was concerned, it was hilarious for him to see me react this way and he could repeat this mockery several times a day. I did not have a good self-esteem. I always felt stupid in everything I said and I thought that I was irrelevant to people. However, at the bottom of my heart, I had this deep conviction that I was intelligent and interesting. But I had a hard time conveying this inner certainty when I got in touch with others.

This unpleasant feeling became stronger when, growing up, my body began to transform itself, when my hips were widening and my thighs and buttocks were becoming rounder. Already, at the age of 12, my body started to displease me. I did not want to experience the

My soul was aware of the fact that the coat wrapping it was not as it should be.

same things as my mother, my grandmother, my aunts and my cousins with regards to my body. I wanted to be comfortable in my own skin and feel like a princess with a dream body. Despite this desire, I was eating and feeling guilty. The more I felt guilty, the more I ate, exceeding the limits of my appetite. I began to develop a feeling of disgust towards my body.

Over the years, my brother kept singing "wonder fatso" to me. He had also added other words that hurt me even more. Furthermore, in high school, I saw that the boys were noticing girls that were slim. Obviously, I did not fit their beauty standards even if I was a beautiful young girl.

Diets

Surely as for many of you, this was the beginning of the diet plans saga. During the first year of high school, I started 3 days diets, diets made exclusively of vegetables, bananas, vegetable soup, cabbage... But the results did not come. I vividly remember putting on a scarf under my sweaters and my swimsuits to tighten my belly and look thinner. I wore firming nylon stockings under my pants. For me, it was unfair that my body would so easily gain weight. I would say: "I hardly eat anything and I gain weight. I just look at chocolate and I get fat..."

Over time, I suffered several disparaging remarks about my weight. At 16 years old, I hated my body. My chubbiness disgusted me. I did not like my nose and several parts of my anatomy. Diets followed in dire succession, one directly after the other. **I lost some of the weight but was constantly gaining it back.** From one mirror to the next, I would watch my body hoping that the next time I would find myself more beautiful. I did not like the image that was reflected. The perception I had of myself was completely distorted and unrealistic.

My Worth

At school, I was always among the first of the class and I excelled in certain sports. After all, I had to take my place and prove to everyone, and especially to myself, that I was worth something, even if I did not like my body. It was a constant challenge for me. I was a perfectionist and consequently, I was brilliantly successful.

How many times have I cried to God to make me lose weight, how often have I shed tears because of this injustice. How often!!!

I desired so much to have a beautiful body, to be gorgeous and feel free with my body. My desire was to wear the beautiful garments I saw in the window displays of the clothing stores. Please do not misunderstand me... I wanted to be slim, happy, and proud of myself for my own satisfaction.

Obsession and Torment

From "Weight Watcher" to proteins and therapies, nothing seemed to improve. Quite the opposite, more time wore on, more I was tormented by this problem. This did not prevent me from performing well in my career. I liked my face, but my well-established excess weight remained a sign of failure. I was managing to control everything in my life except this recurring problem. All the efforts I devoted to losing weight were not producing lasting results.

I attached so much importance to it that I became an expert in nutrition. I knew the calorie count of each food and the content in fiber and fat. I was unbeatable at this game! When I was tired of calculating or of restricting my portions of food, gluttony got the upper hand, and then I would stuff myself.

From complete deprivation to total saturation, I did not know how to feed myself properly without being tormented. My mind tirelessly accounted for everything that I had eaten and all that I was going to eat. It was a constant obsession, and my whole life was devoted to this permanent challenge.

How could I lose weight and keep it off by investing so much effort? How could I hide my distress and this torment to those around me? I went from one extreme to another. I was aware that I couldn't concentrate on anything else.

From Anorexia to Bulimia

When I was 21, the anorexic to bulimic phases began. In a few weeks, I could go from a clothing size of 5 to 14. Sometimes, I emptied my wardrobe, not knowing what to wear. Discouragement followed. I wanted to take nothing but water and ended up in the fridge! I was cancelling all my appointments and invitations because I felt so lousy about myself and too disappointed in myself, suffering emotionally to a degree that I couldn't face up to people.

The worst torment: facing people's judging eyes and their comments. Words like "you put on some weight" were familiar to me. Being accustomed to this reality, I actually did not need to hear them. I was not that big, but I hated my body. I had a poor self-image and was living in guilt and shame. Physical training was not enough. Therapies couldn't break this obsession. Diets did not work... But glory to God! What seemed impossible to me was possible to God and through God.

My Victory!

Today, I live fully my life, without any food restrictions and my body is perfect for me. When people compliment me, I have no other choice but to say thank you and I praise God for what He did. I give Him all the honors I receive from those around me. My body and food made me experience "hell". God has delivered me and God has made me more beautiful. After being slender for ten years without dieting and having gone through two pregnancies, I feel perfectly fine in my body and in my mind.

I would have never imagined that God could and would remove this burden from my life. Through the truth of the Word of God and the revelations received by my husband and myself, the war between food, my soul and my body was finally over! I always say that "a revelation from God brings a revolution in your life"...

Your Victory!

Are you ready to take hold of the 7 keys to live an absolute victory for the well-being of your soul and your body regarding food? **Are you ready** to grasp the freedom with food to which you're entitled? If you're really motivated and you have answered yes to these 2 questions, you will efficiently put into practice the principles contained in this book. You will draw powerful information that you will apply and they will bring tremendous changes in your life.

2. STATISTICS

*A*s a former social worker, I am aware that statistics represent more than numbers: They are really people... Day after day, my job got me to interact with human beings in distress. These percentages hide a more daunting reality, because we know that people with weight and/or eating disorders are ashamed and suffer in silence, thereby withdrawing themselves from the statistics, as I did myself.

> *A statistic is more than a number; it is a human being.*

Here are some statistics that caught my attention:

- An estimated 9 to 10% of adult women suffer from problems related to compulsive eating, including difficulty controlling food intake and an exaggerated attention to weight and shape. (Let's say that I could have been part of this statistic, but nobody knew...)

- No less than 200 scientific studies on the 800 presented at the annual conference of the North American Association for the Study of Obesity (NAASO) are devoted to psychiatric obesity, an alarming phenomenon that affects 12.5 million children and teenagers across the United States. Statistics show that a child with obesity aged between 10 and 14 and with at least one obese parent, is 79% more likely to remain obese as an adult. During childhood, this problem affects more boys (62.7%) than girls (27.8%). In the teenage years, the gap decreases and hovers around 30% for both sexes.

In the United States

- 12% of teenagers aged between 12 and 17 are above their healthy weight.

- 14% of children aged between 6 and 11 are above their healthy weigh.

- It is estimated that some 22 million children aged 5 and under are above their healthy weight.

- 1 in 4 children is above their healthy weight.

- 67% of the North American population is above their healthy weight.

- 20% of North American teenagers are obese.

- 70 to 80% of Americans are above their healthy weight.

In Canada

- The prevalence of obesity increased from 5.6% in 1985 to 14.9% in 2003.

- 80% of women have dieted before age 18.

- 40% of women have dieted before age 9.

- As early as the age of 8 or 9, girls are concerned about their weight!

- 14% of women are overweight.

- 25% of men are overweight.

In Quebec

- An estimated 65,000 young people aged 14 to 25 suffer from eating disorders.

- Today, a quarter of the population aged over 25 is obese and one third is overweight.

- For young people aged 10 to 17, the phenomenon has doubled and intensified in recent years. Obesity increased from 3 to 8% and excess weight, from 12 to 18%.

- 8% of girls aged 15 to 25 are suffering from eating disorders.

- Almost 35% of Quebecers are overweight.

In France

- Obesity is progressing and touching 5.9 million people, nearly twice the numbers of ten years ago. Over 20 million people are overweight.

In Australia

- 51.9% of women are above their healthy weight.

- 67.4% of men are above their healthy weight.[*]

Sources: Statistics Canada (Statistics from 1983 to 2007) - Public Health Agency of Canada - National Population Health Survey, Health Canada - U.S. Government Statistics - World Heart Federation Fact-Sheet, 2002 - Australia's Health 2004, AIHW

More and more young people have very unbalanced eating habits, abuse of diets or medications or are forcing themselves to vomit regularly. They are neither solely bulimic nor solely anorexic, but suffer from atypical disorders of their dietary behaviors.

Starting now, you are in a process of supernatural change. These statistics allow you to see that you are not the only one living the problems of obesity and/or eating disorders. The numbers speak for themselves! You have become aware of them. Throughout the pages of this book, you will change; you will be transformed both inwardly and outwardly. In time, you will no longer be part of these statistics, but of the Army of God that is getting up! You have the strength and the power of God in your life.

3. COMMITMENT CONTRACT

*T*o achieve an absolute victory, I invite you to immediately take action and to take a step forward by filling out the following contract of commitment. *Psalms 50:14b-15* says:

> *"... pay thy vows unto the Most High: And call upon me in the day of trouble: I will deliver thee, and thou shalt glorify me."*

Make a commitment before God and honor it! If you do your part, God will do the rest. Your life will change forever. This will be the foundation of your complete victory, and you will see your desire to be free and slim come true. God is able to deliver you and lift you up. Not only is He able to, but He wants to!!!

When we make a commitment to God, and stick to this decision, we can see that the Lord is faithful to His word to bring us victory. Furthermore, when we write our goals and keep them in front of our eyes, it is proven that the success rate is increased to 98%. While keeping the contract in front of you, imagine what your potential for success will be... I can tell you that it will be a 100% success rate! Partnering with God is always a source of victories!

Be **Free**, Be **Slim**!

7 Keys
to Total Victory
Over Food and Your Body

I, _____ , hereby pledge to :

- Put my contract within sight.
- Read and re-read several times a week each key discussed in this book.
- Apply the spiritual teachings I received, as reflected in the implementation, in order to integrate them into my personal life.
- Repeat aloud as often as possible the prayers and verses given in the book.

I recognize that God does not lie in his Word and that He desires for me:

- To be well in my body.
- To be free in my relationship with food.
- To be healthy.
- To be slim.
- To be beautiful/handsome.

Write your personal goals in relation to food and your body:

- _____
- _____
- _____
- _____

In witness whereof, I have signed on this ____ day of the month of _____ in the year 20__.

4. DOES GOD WANT AND CAN MAKE ME BE FREE AND SLIM?

*P*eople often say: "Ah! If it is God's will, He will do this or that for me..." Well, I can assure you that the Word of God is clear on several specific points concerning the will of the Father for His children. All we need is to be aware about it through the knowledge of the Bible, to want it and claim it. In fact, God's will is for us to be prospering in every aspect, in all areas of our lives, including our physical, emotional and psychological freedom regarding food.

> *"Beloved, I wish above all things that thou mayest **prosper and be in health**, even **as thy soul prospereth.**"*
>
> *3 John 1:2*

God is a God of love who wants to see His children blossom and be happy in all aspects of their lives. If you are tormented by food, dieting and the appearance of your body (too skinny, too fat, too...), it is certainly not God's will for you!

When I teach people that are overweight and/or tormented with food, I often repeat this: "It's not your weight on the scale that matters, it's how good you feel in your body." For some, a weight of 160 pounds (73 kg) is correct. For many, 120 pounds (55 kg) on the scale is ideal, for others it's 105 pounds (48 kg). The number on the scale is irrelevant. What matters the most is this: "How do you feel?" Are you at ease or uneasy when you go out in public? Are you embarrassed when you make love? Is it hard for you to climb stairs or to run? Are you uncomfortable when you sit in your car? If the answer is yes to any of these questions, the next lines will be of particular interest to you.

Everything God Has Created is Perfect

I have a perfect God of love who creates all things with love. Knowing this, I was wondering why some people were sometimes being afflicted with an imperfect body, some infirmity, or disease.

On a beautiful morning of prayer, I asked the Lord why some children were born with disabilities and health issues. As a mother touched by children and their happiness, I couldn't conceive that God would send sick or disabled children in certain families. Is there anything these parents need to learn? Are these children examples for others, models of determination and courage?

When the Lord answered me, the explanation was simpler than I thought. God said: "Everything I create is perfect, flawless, and fashioned with beauty. All my works are marvelous and magnificent. Nothing I do is imperfect. I am a perfect God who does everything perfectly. It is sin that brought curses in the world, and it now affects my creation's health, body, and success. This is what brings destruction and imperfection."

God always lays a perfect seed in a woman's body. She then unites with the seed of a man. If the soil is rich and fertile, the baby will be born in good condition. Adversely, if the generational land is in poor condition (for example: grandparents and parents that have sinned), there is a possibility this child will be subjected "unfairly" to this legacy transmitted through his/her bloodline. We all come from different "soils" through our bloodline. Sometimes they are very well looked after by faith and the Word of God, while at other times, not in the least!

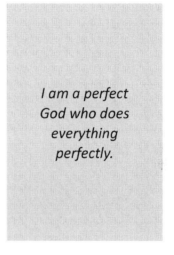

I am a perfect God who does everything perfectly.

To end this, it is essential to break this generational curse in the name of Jesus Christ.

God said: "I sent my only Son Jesus Christ to redeem the world from the curse. He became a curse so that you are no longer under the curse. All those who have accepted my only Son as Savior and Lord do not have to pay this price in their lives. Sin no longer reigns in their bodies. They are no longer under the curse of the law and sin, but under grace, forgiven and washed. They have become new creations. All I create is perfect, including children in their mother's womb. The curse that pervades in the world affects and sometimes destroys my creation. However, I gave my children the authority to reject all curses and to live the abundant life for which my Son paid the price at the cross. Just believe, believe in my Word and receive it."

*"For God so loved the world that **He gave His only begotten Son, that whosoever believeth in him should not perish**, but have everlasting life."*

John 3:16

*"**Christ hath redeemed us from the curse of the law**, being made a curse for us: for it is written, Cursed is everyone that hangeth on a tree."*

Galatians 3:13

*"The thief cometh not, but for to steal, and to kill, and to destroy: **I am come** that they might have life, and **that they might have it more abundantly**."*

John 10:10

*"I call heaven and earth to record this day against you, that I have set before you life and death, blessing and cursing: therefore **choose life, that both thou and thy seed may live**."*

Deuteronomy 30:19

The Devil Wants to Destroy God's Creation

In the beginning, God created us free, slim and healthy.

God does not want our bodies to be destroyed. If anyone wants to destroy God's creation, it is our enemy: the devil. That's why people are carrying generational curses and the child that comes into the world unintentionally "inherits" this spiritual weight. The following principle is important to understand. When we become children of God by giving our lives to Jesus Christ, we have the authority to break all generational curses that were prevalent in our bloodline. We will address this later.

It is so reassuring to know that Jesus Christ redeemed us from all curses and that He gave us the power to reject them from our lives. Hallelujah! In the beginning, God created us free, slim and healthy. When you become a child of God, you have the privilege to repossess the real life for which you were created.

> *"If you, then, though you are evil, know how to give good gifts to your children, **how much more will your Father in heaven give good gifts to those who ask him.**"*
>
> *Matthew 7:11*

God wants us:

- To be prosper in every aspect (including our relationship with food and our body).
- To feel very good in our body at all times.
- To have enough breath to climb the stairs.
- To love ourselves in the clothes that we wear.
- To increase our personal dignity.
- To feel great anytime, anywhere and in any occasion.
- To keep our body healthy, holy and perfect in God's image.
- To have a body free from overweight.
- To be in shape, serene and happy.
- To have all the energy necessary to accomplish the work for which He has destined us.
- To eat nutritious and balanced food.
- To take care of our body: the temple of the Holy Spirit.
- To be balanced, constant and persistent in everything we do.
- To achieve success in all our businesses.
- To be stable and disciplined.
- To grant us the desires of our heart.
- To reflect the glory of God when people look at us.

God does not want us:

- To be filled with self-hatred.
- To live in constant dissatisfaction.
- To be slaves to food.
- To be tormented by food and/or our weight.
- To have difficulty getting out of bed, getting up from the car seat, putting on pants that became too small…
- To be on a diet the rest of our lives.
- To worry excessively about our weight.
- To be restricted.
- To fluctuate from one extreme to another.
- To develop health problems due to obesity or being underweight.**

God wants his people to walk in the blessing. The blessing means to be clothed with the power to prosper. You received the power to prosper, including prosperity for your body. The extension of the blessing is the result. The result of the blessing will allow you to have a healthy and beautiful body, in the original state that God has created it.

If you want to **become a child of God** *and experience all the benefits of His salvation in your life, read and repeat aloud the* **prayer of repentance** *in the appendix on page 272.*

**Sources: Ps. 20:5-6, Matt. 5:4, Ps. 28:6-7, Gal. 3:13, Ps. 37:4, Gal. 3:29, Ps. 61:6, 1 Cor. 3:17, Ps. 139:13-16, Heb. 6:12, Isa. 30:18, 3 Jn. 1:2, Isa. 54:4-5, 2 Pe. 2:19.

Fearfully and Wonderfully Made

*"I will praise thee; for **I am fearfully and wonderfully made**: marvelous are thy works; and that my soul knoweth right well."*

Psalms 139.14

Several years ago, these four words have become a revelation for me. I am wonderfully made… How much of an effect they had on my soul! The Word of God was totally contrary to the multitude of negative words that I had received since my youth. Most of the time, I did not love myself. I did not like my body. I was always comparing myself with other women and felt I rarely measured up.

It was on a Sunday morning while I was praising the Lord in church that verse 14 of Psalm 139 was brought back to my mind. I began to speak it with conviction over myself. One day, God made me realize that he loved me so much and that He really wanted me to feel good in my body. God wanted me to integrate this powerful revelation so that I could receive His word: **I am wonderfully made!**

"I am come that they might have life, and that they might have it more abundantly."

John 10:10

I then asked Him to forgive me for having despised myself so much.

The thief that came to steal my dignity and my self-esteem, who wanted to destroy my body was called Satan. He used people around me. This certainly was not the will of God that I hate my body and **His** creation. How could I praise God for being such a wonderful creation when I hated myself so, when I was so utterly dissatisfied with my body? Then God made me understand that He had created me to be beautiful and to be proud of His handiwork. In reality, it was none other than myself! There and then I asked Him to forgive me for having despised myself so much. I asked him to see myself through His eyes so I could take back what the thief had stolen from me without my knowledge.

Satan had robbed me for too long... Years and years of living with overweight, developing eating disorders. I always heard this small voice that kept telling me that I would never be slim. I was conditioning myself to live with a weight surplus since all the women in my family were corpulent, bordering on being obese. The thief made me believe that the problem was running in the family, that I would always have to be careful about what I eat and that I would be dieting all my life. Blah-blah…

Satan is a liar! What he says is only deception. He lures the world with his lies to keep God's creation bound. The divine truth is otherwise. The Lord has a perfect plan for me. The Word of God is beyond the falsehoods of Satan.

The wisdom of God is foolishness to man. The Word of God reveals to me that I am a **new creation**, old things are passed away. I am the progeny of Abraham through Jesus Christ. He has redeemed me from the curse. He came to give me life in abundance, that I succeed with everything I undertake. I am fearfully and wonderfully made, a marvelous creation indeed. Glory to God!

> ***"Therefore if any man be in Christ, he is a new creature:*** *old things are passed away; behold, all things are become new."*
> *2 Corinthians 5:17*

> *"And if ye be Christ's, then are ye Abraham's seed, and heirs according to the promise."*
> *Galatians 3:29*

I decided to exercise my power of decision to go and get the promises that God had for me with unwavering resolve. I did not accept Satan's lies. It was out of the question that I pay the price for past generations and accept the curse on women's bodies in my bloodline... No thanks!

Jesus Christ Paid THE Price

> *"Surely he took up our pain and bore our suffering, yet we considered him punished by God, stricken by him, and afflicted"*
>
> *Isaiah 53:4*
> *(Today's New International Version)*

Bring your attention to these powerful words from the Word of God. Jesus Christ bore our suffering... But what is the suffering? Have you taken the time to reflect on the meaning of this word? The dictionary defines the word "suffering" as the state of feeling physical or moral pain, to be tormented by and injured by…

If you suffer from eating disorders, **if you suffer** psychologically about food and/or your weight, **if you suffer** from being overweight and/or hatred towards your body, give it all to the Lord! Surrender yourself completely!

He paid THE price for you. He bore your sufferings. He carried your physical and psychological hurts and pains. Hallelujah!

Jesus Christ paid THE price for you to have a life of abundance, joy, and blessings. Not so you can "look" happy on Sunday morning in church. No! The Lord desires that you really be serene and well with yourself. It is time to integrate this biblical truth in your life: you are fearfully and wonderfully made!

> *"But he was wounded for our transgressions, he was bruised for our iniquities: the chastisement of our peace was upon him; and with his stripes we are healed."*
>
> *Isaiah 53:5*

Receive Complete Salvation

Why would you pay for something that has already been paid for you? Jesus Christ bore the punishment so we can be at peace: at peace when you eat, at peace towards your body, at peace in your mind, at

The world's mindset is to believe that we must always fight with the same problem and that we must absolutely go on a diet to loose weight.

peace with your emotions, at peace ALL THE TIME. The world's mindset is to believe that we must always fight with the same problem and it is absolutely necessary to diet to loose weight. **The world's mindset is contrary to the mind of God.** It is foreign to God's wisdom. You do not have to "accept" the curse on your body.

Choose to receive the complete salvation for which Jesus Christ has paid THE price. Choose to take back by force peace and absolute victory in your life. God wants us healthy and full of energy, feeling good in our body, beautiful because He creates all things to be beautiful, sometimes on the fringe of convention, but still beautiful! He did not call imperfect things into existence. He does everything perfectly.

Satan takes pleasure to undo, to destroy the wonderful works of our God. However, the Lord is stronger than anything. Glory to God!

"for everyone born of God overcomes the world. This is the victory that has overcome the world, even our faith."

1 John 5:4

"Jesus looked at them and said, "With man this is impossible, but with God all things are possible."

Matthew 19:26

"I can do everything through him who gives me strength."

Philippians 4:13

HALLELUJAH!

After reading the previous lines, take a few minutes and ask the Lord for forgiveness for having perhaps despised yourself at one or several occasions. Release the Word of God upon yourself, believing you are created in his image and that you are fearfully and wonderfully made, a marvelous creation indeed.

And God said: "Let us make man in our image, after our likeness: and let them have dominion over the fish of the sea, and over the fowl of the air, and over the cattle, and over all the earth, and over every creeping thing that creepeth upon the earth."

Genesis 1:26

Be Free, Be Slim!

Rejoice and know that you are about to see the realization of your desire to be free and slim. God is able to deliver you and uplift you! Not only is He able to, He wants to! I rejoice because it is the beginning of the end of these torments!

This is the start of a new life for you. The more you apply the principles contained in this book, the greater your opportunity of success will be. Be perseverant! I repeat: if you do your part, God will support you and do the rest. Never forget that the wisdom of the world is not the wisdom of God. Devote all your attention to the Word of the Eternal God rather than listening to Satan's lies. He has stolen enough of your energy, your time, and your life by tormenting you in a thousand and one ways. It's enough!

> *Rejoice and know that you are about to see the realization of your desire to be free and slim.*

50

Applying the Principles

1. Discard or hide your scale. What matters is not the weight on the scale; it is your well-being.

2. Reduce (or stop altogether) the time you spend watching TV shows related to fashion and do this for a few weeks. Avoid reading magazines that may bring you to compare your weight and appearance with models whose photos were retouched by computer.

3. Pray these words as often as possible:

   Lord Jesus,

   I know you are the Son of God and that you gave your life so that I might be saved. I ask your forgiveness for everything I have done in the past and I give my life to you. Become the Savior and Lord of my life. I ask your forgiveness for each time I hated myself, that I looked in the mirror and judged the work of your hands, which is my body. Starting today, please allow me to see myself as you see me. I give you all my sufferings, including my discomfort related to food and my body.

I receive Your Peace, the true peace from you. I declare that I,

(your name) _____,

am fearfully and wonderfully made, a marvelous creation indeed.

In the name of Jesus Christ. Amen!

4. Repeat this verse aloud three times a day, every day for the next 7 weeks: "I am fearfully and wonderfully made." Your thoughts about yourself will be renewed by the Word of God through your mouth.

5. Always remember that God's wisdom is foolishness to man. Always question yourself by asking the following: "Do I have God's thoughts about this situation or the thoughts of man?"

5. YOUR BODY CANNOT BE MORE PROSPEROUS THAN YOUR SOUL

"Beloved, I wish above all things that thou mayest prosper and be in health, even as thy soul prospereth."

3 John 1:2

This verse is clear: It is God's will that we prosper in all respects. This means at all levels, in all areas of our lives, including our psychological, emotional and physical freedom.

Your body's beauty is the extension of the prosperity of your soul.

God does not want us to live in constant torment regarding our body and food. He does not want us to suffer from eating disorders or complexes about our body. We are such wonderful creations!

God wants us to prosper as our soul prospers. The Word of God is clear: to be in abundance, everything is played in the realm of the soul. What you have in your life is the blessing of God and the demonstration of the prosperity of your soul.

But What is the Soul?

The soul consists of your emotions, your thoughts, your personality and your will. Your thoughts must be prosperity-oriented to receive abundance in your life. **The same is true** for your emotions and your will. Your soul must be strengthened by the power of the Holy Spirit so that all be accomplished.

The Relationship Between Your Soul and Your Slenderness

Assuming that the state of your soul is what prospers you. You must understand that the fight for complete victory over food and your slenderness is primarily happening in your mind. Your soul (your mind, will and emotions) is the war zone.

Satan's war zone really was in my thoughts, but he was also playing with my emotions.

Previously, when I was trying all sorts of ways to lose weight, I realized that the problem was not losing the weight; it was stabilizing it once I had reached my objective. I was seeing my body shrink but over time, "I was playing Yo-Yo." Reflecting on all this, I told myself: "My body is not the real problem, since I'm able to lose the weight; it is my way of thinking that's erroneous." I was not wrong.

One of Satan's Strategies

We must understand that Satan sows thoughts and waits to see whether we will accept them or not. He is the tempter and the accuser *(Revelation 11:10)*. If we bite on the bait and fall, he just "gained more ground". He then gives himself a "legal territory" in the life of that person and can now bring her to her own destruction. Subsequently, he torments that person day and night, putting accusatory thoughts in her mind: "It's your fault; you're no good." Satan affects the person's soul so he can destroy her prosperity. Anyone who has eating disorders and/or weight issues has inevitably been affected by the enemy in their emotions, thoughts and will. Overeating first arises in the thoughts, emotions, and will. This is an extension of what happens in the soul. Satan is the father of lies and injects false thoughts to have an impact on people's lives. Remember he is a thief, a destroyer, and a murderer *(John 10:10)*.

Our Soul is Not Born Again, It is Renewed

When we are born again and become a child of God, we are a new creation. Our spirit is born again, but not our soul. **We must work to renew our thoughts and emotions according to the Word of God so that our soul can be transformed and become prosperous in keeping with the will of God.** The more we saturate ourselves with the presence of the Lord, the more we read the Word of God, and the more we will know The Truth.

*"And be not conformed to this world: **but be ye transformed by the renewing of your mind**, that ye may prove what is that good, and acceptable, and perfect, will of God."*

Romans 12:2

"And ye shall know the truth and the truth shall make you free."

John 8:32

Understanding the truth is what makes us free. To be free, our intelligence, our thoughts must be renewed through the Word of God. But free from what? Have you ever asked yourself this question? Are you only spiritually free? No! You are free in all areas of your life! Anyhow, when we are spiritually free, when our soul receives and comprehends a revelation from the Word of God, it has no choice but to be freed in the natural realm as well.

Your relationship with food as well as with your body needs to be freed by the Word of God!

Everything happens in the realm of your soul. The 7 keys that follow will allow you to unlock the prosperity your soul needs so that you can be truly free and slim!

Your Soul is Like a Body

Your soul is like a body that has many muscles. Some muscles are stronger and others, weaker. We need to work out harder on the weaker muscles to make them stronger.

We can draw a parallel between them and certain areas of your life. Sometimes, this "muscle" is weaker and it is necessary to be more rigorous in this specific area of your life so you can develop and strengthen it. You may realize in your life that other areas (muscles) are stronger. You are successful and things are easy for you. Now, in this same area, that which is very easy for you can be very difficult for someone else.

Your soul is stronger at this level and you do not need to be so rigorous... It's easy! Yet for the other, it is not. The reverse is true as well. Many people may feel very strong in a particular area, while for you it is your "muscular" weakness!

Are you longing for a "normal life" with food and your slenderness? Do you want to be like those who are naturally slim and who claim to be able to eat everything they want without putting on weight? What can you learn from them? The answer is simple: they have no fear related to food and their bodies. This area of their soul is muscular. From now on, to obtain the same results as those people, you must be rigorous so you may strengthen this "muscle" of your soul.

You must not conform (imitate) to these present times anymore. You are new creations transformed by what the Word of God says about you. What I find interesting is that the word "transformed" comes from the Greek word "metamorphoo", which means undergoing a METAMORPHOSIS. What a powerful word! To undergo a metamorphosis, we must be renewed in our mind (soul).

For your body to be transformed and for you to live a free life for which Jesus Christ paid the price at the cross, you must be renewed in your mind. This "muscle" of your soul must be

To undergo a metamorphosis, we must be renewed in our mind (soul).

strengthened by the renewing of your thoughts and a new programming regarding food and your body. This part of your soul has been fed with lies as: "Ah! It's hard to lose weight... I can't help it; I'm like my mother... I took medications and now I'm paying the price for it, etc..."

Starting today, you must strengthen that part of your soul through the Word of God, which is the truth. You are not like the world anymore. Your soul must now be renewed so it can see things like God sees them. Seeing things and talking like the world is over. The more you fill yourself up with the truth of God and His presence, the more your personality, your emotions and your thoughts change from glory to glory. You

58

can decide to begin a new weight loss program or the next best therapy to be free from eating disorders. It's your choice!

> *However, if you are looking for a real,*
> *unique and lasting solution, there's only one:*
> *the Truth of the Word of God*
> *applied diligently in your life.*

Your soul must see itself slim so that you can become slim. It must perceive itself the way God sees things. **To be free and slim, you must feed your soul with the truth of the Word of God.**

Be Strong My Soul!

For your soul to see itself free and slim, you have to strengthen it. You must train it to strengthen itself. The training consists in speaking aloud to it as David was doing with his own soul. Throughout his moments of weakness, he did not let himself be pulled down by this state. He was literally speaking to his soul and releasing God's truth over it.

> *"Why art thou cast down, O my soul? and why art thou disquieted in me? hope thou in God: for I shall yet praise him for the help of his countenance."*
>
> *Psalms 42:6*

59

When some days are harder and you feel like quitting and going back to bed, do the contrary! Confront your soul (your thoughts, your emotions, your will) with the Word of God through your mouth. When you look at yourself in the mirror and the enemy tries to play with your thoughts, do not get involved in his game. Speak to your soul and repeat what the Word of God says about you: you are fearfully and wonderfully made, a marvelous creation indeed, you are the head and not the tail, you are a descendant of Abraham and Sarai through Jesus Christ, etc.

Put your hands on your chest, where your emotions are located, and say, "Soul, you will be strengthened in the name of Jesus Christ! Why do you pull yourself down? The Word of God says you are fearfully and wonderfully made, a marvelous creation..." The more we muscle ourselves spiritually, the more we can be amazed at how effective and powerful these teachings are.

"So shall my word be that goeth forth out of my mouth: it shall not return unto me void, but it shall accomplish that which I please, and it shall prosper in the thing whereto I sent it."
Isaiah 55:11

Applying the Principles

1. Satan's war zone is in your soul: your thoughts, your emotions, and your will.

2. Remember that your soul must strengthen itself (muscled itself) so that your body can experience an absolute victory and your relationship with food be transformed once and for all.

3. Work to renew your mind in this area of your life according to the Word of God, in order for you to be truly free and slim!

4. Speak to your soul as often as possible so that it can become stronger, more "muscled" and achieve real and sustainable results.

Section Two

THE ROOTS OF THE PROBLEM

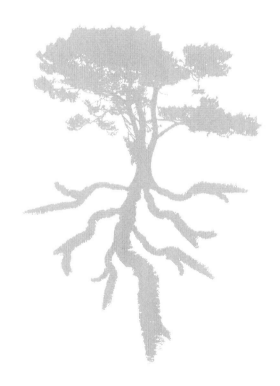

"Identify the true root of the problem so you may confront it and conquer it."

The Roots of the Problem

*I*n this second section, you will discover the **one** or **many** roots of the problem coming against your relationship with food and/or against your body. **To solve a problem, you must absolutely identify its source. The quicker you pinpoint the root of the problem, the quicker the victory will come.**

Most of the time, people languish in the same situation, the same problem, the same "pattern" for the longest time. They have not clearly identified the root of the problem and/or simply because they did not identify and did not confront it. Discouragement follows. You can no longer recognize the real cause of this torment. Therefore, you cannot overturn this painful situation and come out victorious. Perhaps you've tried all sorts of ways to overcome these issues of surplus weight and/or torment with food, hoping to see your body transform itself miraculously? Unfortunately, your attempts proved to be unsuccessful and probably without lasting effect.

Rejoice! In the next pages, you will discover the root of your problem. With the 7 keys I will give you in section three, you'll be able to overcome and emerge victorious from this battle. Please understand me: if you identify the exact root of the problem that is coming against you and you confront it with the appropriate methods, the right principles and keys, you will surely obtain the victory. It is certain! There are 7 possible roots and one or several of them can be the source of your problem. Take the time to identify the true root of your problem so you can destroy it forever.

Let's now use a problem tree as an example. It bears bad fruits. This tree is a problem in your life. It grows because it originates from a **seed** that grows **roots**, and then a **trunk**, **branches** and **leaves**.

When we want to destroy a problem tree, it has to be done from the roots. We must burn the roots of this tree to make them die. The more you will go to the source, the foundation of the problem, the more you will be able to make it disappear. If we try to eliminate a tree by cutting only the trunk, this tree will most assuredly grow back. Of course, it will no longer be visible to the naked eye, but this is only an illusion. It will only last for a short while. The more you will try to eliminate this tree by cutting down the trunk, the stronger it will grow back in your life.

If we compare this tree to your dietary freedom and your body, **you proceeded the same way**. For years, you wanted to remove this tree (this problem) from your sight (your life). You've tried for years to cut this tree from the trunk, i.e. through countless diets and trying to control what you eat. The only thing you produced in your life is a short bout of slenderness, and then, you probably saw the problem grow wider and stronger. This is called the "Yo-Yo" or "accordion" phenomenon.

In other cases, some people seem to have solved the weight issue. They lost some of it, but the tree grew back in other ways. It is still there, but it in a different fashion. They are slim, but tormented about food. They are afraid to be overweight again; they eat little, constantly restrain themselves and develop eating disorders. Finally, they are not really free: the tree is still there.

To permanently remove the tree, you must go to the main root, which is spiritual and not carnal. Through this second section you will, at last, identify the root of the root itself. Glory to God! How, several years ago, would I have loved to know about the principles that I am teaching you now. You also, I imagine! How much time we could have saved! How much suffering we would have been spared from!

> *"For we wrestle not against flesh and blood, but against principalities, against powers, against the rulers of the darkness of this world, against spiritual wickedness in high places."*
>
> *Ephesians 6:12*

FIRST ROOT:

Generational Curses

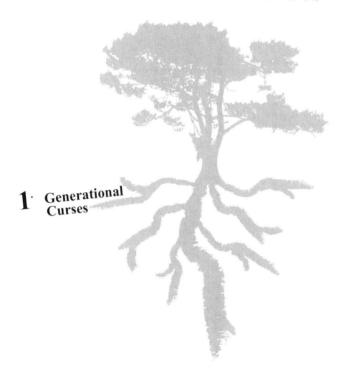

1· Generational Curses

It is simple to see whether one of the root of your problem comes from your bloodline. You only have to look at your extended family: parents, grandpa-

It is the case of 75% of the people having eating disorders or chronic obesity.

rents, siblings, cousins, aunts, and uncles... If you find that it is a recurring problem in your family, it is most likely one of the roots that unwittingly brought this curse in your life. You did not deserve it...

In families where we find this generational curse, it can come under different guises. For example:

- People are overweight since their childhood.
- People start to be overweight in their teenage years (it was my case).
- Women suffer from obesity after one or more pregnancies.
- Women are overweight at menopause.
- Men are overweight after their thirties, in their forties, and fifties.

If you notice the same "pattern" in your bloodline, this is certainly a generational curse.

However and fortunately, when we become a child of God, we no longer have to undergo and live with generational curses in our bloodline. When Jesus Christ came, He redeemed us from all curses.

> *"Christ hath redeemed us from the curse of the law, being made a curse for us: for it is written, Cursed is every one that hangeth on a tree."*
> *Galatians 3:13*

"And if ye be Christ's, then are ye Abraham's seed, and heirs according to the promise."

Galatians 3:29

My DNA changed

Since I am now a descendant of Abraham through Jesus Christ, I receive the blessing that was on my "spiritual father and mother", Abraham and Sarai.

And Scripture, foreseeing that God would justify the Gentiles through faith, foretold this good news to Abraham:

"And if ye be Christ's, then are ye Abraham's seed, and heirs according to the promise."

Galatians 3:29

"In thee shall all nations be blessed. So then they which be of faith are blessed with faithful Abraham."

Galatians 3:8-9

Note that the blessing is for those who believe. **What you believe is what you receive.**

If you believe you will experience the same thing as your bloodline, you will receive exactly that. However, if you believe what the Word of God says – that your bloodline has changed through Jesus Christ – it is what you will receive.

Hallelujah! Remember that it is the truth that sets us free *(John 8:32)* and that truth comes from the Word of God.

The Word of God is clear and precise about the fact that we have become new creations and that old things have passed away.

> *"Therefore if any man be in Christ, he is a new creature: old things are passed away; behold, all things are become new."*
>
> 2 Corinthians 5:17

I am then the seed of Abraham... Every born again child of God becomes the seed of Abraham and heir to the promise. But what promise? The promise that Abraham's descendants would enjoy the same blessings that God had bestowed to Abraham and his wife Sarai. What a gift! God is so good! Therefore, curses that were on my earthly family are not handed down to me anymore, but I inherit the blessing that was on the life of my "spiritual father and mother", Abraham and Sarai.

From the Invisible to the Visible

Do you think the blessing remains in the invisible, the supernatural, and makes no difference in your life on this earth? The power of the blessing brings total transformation to your life to provide you with the best. The blessing takes from the invisible to the visible what God has in store for you.

70

What is the advantage of learning that our bloodline has changed? When I looked closer at "my spiritual bloodline", I saw that Sarai was simply a gorgeous woman, as were her descendants: Rebekah, Rachel…

> *"And it came to pass, when he was come near to enter into Egypt, that he said unto **Sarai** his wife, Behold now, I know that thou art a fair woman to look upon: Therefore it shall come to pass, when the Egyptians shall see thee, that they shall say, This is his wife: and they will kill me, but they will save thee alive. Say, I pray thee, thou art my sister: that it may be well with me for thy sake; and my soul shall live because of thee. And it came to pass, that, when Abram was come into Egypt, **the Egyptians beheld the woman that she was very fair.**"*
>
> *Genesis 12:11-14*

> *"Before he had finished speaking, behold, out came **Rebekah**, who was the daughter of Bethuel son of Milcah, who was the wife of Nahor the brother of Abraham, with her water jar on her shoulder. And the girl **was very beautiful and attractive, chaste and modest**, and unmarried. And she went down to the well, filled her water jar, and came up."*
>
> *Genesis 24:15-16 (Amplified Bible)*

*"Leah was tender eyed; but **Rachel was beautiful and well favoured.**"*

Genesis 29:17

Reading this story carefully, we realize Sarai was not in the prime of her life. She was in her late sixties. Imagine for a moment… The King wanted her for him when he could have been attracted to a multitude of young girls. Sarai was visibly a very beautiful woman. God had chosen her for Abraham, just as he had given Job the three most beautiful daughters in the land (*Job 42:15*). Esther was chosen as a queen among all the other young girls in the land *(Esther 2:17)*. God's will is that we be marvelous creations, and feel good about ourselves as much as Sarai, Rachel and Esther did.

Considering all this, you do not have to accept the curse that came on your body as a consequence of past generations. Your DNA has changed, and you now enjoy the blessing that was on Sarai of being strong and handsome if you are a man, or beautiful and slender if you are a woman. You reflect the glory of God. You become charismatic, possessing great inner, and outer beauty. Others will perceive this difference in you.

You inherit The Blessing. This blessing brings prosperity, favor, health, success, beauty... All the legacy of the curse (physical, emotional, and financial problems) of your biological parents no longer exists. Such was my case. The issues of obesity from past generations will disappear from your life, just as they did in mine. If you are born again in Jesus Christ, your legacy is now that of Sarai's: to be an exceptionally beautiful woman or a very handsome man.

Satan Hates Beauty

Religiosity has often led us to believe that one must be humble and not fixated on one's appearance. Referring to the scriptures, we can see that we must have humility before God. Our hearts must be humble before the Lord and not be filled with pride for what we are or what we possess. In fact, humility is to fear the Lord and continually obey Him. It is God who blesses us so He may be glorified, not for us to take the glory for ourselves. Take time to thank God for everything He has done in your life.

Concerning looks, it is a lie from the pit to think that beauty is not important to God. When we observe all that God created, we

> *When we observe all that God created, we see that He has done so with striking beauty.*

see that He has done so with beauty. Look at nature, landscapes, flowers, babies... We can see the glory of God reflected in everything He created. **Satan hates beauty... Do you know why? Because he was thrown out of the Kingdom of God and lost all his beauty.** Did you know that God had created him as the most beautiful angel?

*"Thou sealest up the sum, full of wisdom, and **perfect in beauty.**"*

Ezekiel 28:12b

*"**Thine heart was lifted up because of thy beauty**, thou hast corrupted thy wisdom by reason **of thy brightness**: I will cast thee to the ground, I will lay thee before kings, that they may behold thee. Thou hast defiled thy sanctuaries by the multitude of thine iniquities, by the iniquity of thy traffick; therefore will I bring forth a fire from the midst of thee, it shall devour thee, and I will bring thee to ashes upon the earth in the sight of all them that behold thee."*

Ezekiel 28:17-18

Satan, who was called Lucifer before his rebellion, was created with astonishing beauty, but because his heart got filled with pride, he lost everything, including his beauty.

"Before destruction the heart of man is haughty, and before honour is humility."

Proverbs 18:12

Satan Wants to Destroy Beauty

As you embellish, know how to recognize the work of God upon you and glorify the Lord.

Satan was destroyed by the fire of God's wrath. It is the all-consuming fire of God. He lost all his shimmer, splendor and beauty. That's why he hates beauty. He wants to destroy everything

God creates with such beauty and rob God's children of all splendor. Moreover, it is no coincidence if among God's people, most people do not feel good about themselves and know consciously or unconsciously they are not at their maximum potential.

Reject once and for all this lie from your adversary, the devil. Show him the manifestation of the glory of God in your body by asserting your beauty. Do not make the same mistake as Satan, which is taking this glory for you. As you embellish, know how to recognize the work of God upon you and glorify the Lord. Hallelujah!

You do not have one minute to lose. Go get a hold of your promises! The promise to you is that you are a child of God, and the progeny of Abraham. Your DNA has changed. Genes and the blood flowing through you now come from the royal blood of Jesus Christ. His blood is pure, without flaws. His blood heals, restores, and transforms.

> *Today, consciously receive the DNA of a child of God.*

Say This Prayer:

Father,

You have given me your DNA. All the sins of past generations have left my life. And as you have ordered, I receive my real spiritual DNA in my soul and in my body, saying that I am now a new creation in Jesus Christ.

I am born again from the incorruptible seed of the Word of God.

(1 Peter 1:23)

I am the light of this world, and I remain in the light.

(Ephesians 5:8)

I am cleansed of all sins, I remove every sin from my life, and I receive forgiveness.

(Romans 13:12, Psalms 104:2)

I am love because you are love and by faith, I loose the love for myself and my body.

(Romans 13:9, 1 John 2:9-11, 3:14)

I am a new creature. The old things are now over. Everything concerning me has changed.
(2 Corinthians 5:17)

I expect to see the glory of God manifested in myself and my body (John 17:10) because I have received my new spiritual DNA!

In the name of Jesus Christ. Amen!

SECOND ROOT :

Your Spouse

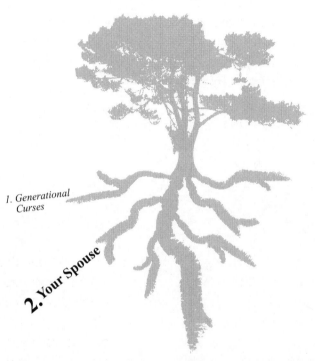

1. Generational Curses

2. Your Spouse

*"And said, For this cause shall a man leave father and mother, and shall cleave to his wife: and **they twain shall be one flesh? Wherefore they are no more twain, but one flesh.** What therefore God hath joined together, let not man put asunder."*

Matthew 19:5-6

When You Become a Couple, You Become "One" Spiritually.

I noticed that several people did not have any weight problem before being a couple. When they met their overweight spouse, they began to get heavier without changing their eating habits and/or daily activities. The best example I can give is when my husband Allen met me. He had never been overweight in all his life. The problem did not exist in his family either. He was training 4 to 5 days per week at the gym and had a muscular body without excess fat.

What was coming against my body had an influence on his own body.

However, when we became a couple and had our first sexual intercourse, he began to gain weight and show some belly fat. He couldn't understand this... He would say: "It makes no sense! I have not changed the way I'm eating. I train several times a week and I'm gaining weight!" He was right... He had not changed a single thing in the natural. But in the spiritual, it was quite another matter. He was now "One" with me.

What was coming against my body had an influence on his body. Not being able to tap into the spiritual knowledge and teachings we possess today, he managed to get rid of this annoyance. How? He adamantly refused this problem in his life by saying: "I've never had a weight problem in my life and I will not have one now. That's enough!"

You must understand that he refused to yield to the spirit that came against me, and now came after him. He did not let himself be pressured. If this is your case, you must take action in the same way Allen did.

It is no coincidence if you start to feel new emotions and have new reactions resembling those of your spouse when you become "One" with him or her.

I often hear people say:

- I get angry more easily than before since I've been with this person...
- I started to have anxiety attacks since I've been married to that person...
- I have trouble with my finances since I've been living with this person. I've never experienced these problems before. I don't understand!

This is very easy to understand. It is indeed written in the Word of God that marriage causes two people to become "One" and the ensuing sexual relation produces unity in the spiritual. This also means that whatever comes spiritually against your spouse also tries to come against you because you're now one and same flesh. The person who has never been through an anxiety attack begins to experience them because the other partner has this problem, etc. But beware! It is important to understand that your refusal has precedence over this spiritual influence and like Allen, you can take authority over this spirit and cast it out of your life.

> *You can take authority over this spirit and cast it out of your life.*

Say This Prayer:

Lord Jesus,

I thank you, for you have freed me from all curses.

I refuse to pay the price of the curse of being overweight that is on my spouse. I do not bear this curse on my life nor my body.

Unclean spirit, I refuse your presence in my life and I command you to leave me immediately in the name of Jesus Christ. I forbid you to return in my life. I've cast you out, and you will remain out.

I now proclaim that my body gets back to its original shape.

In the name of Jesus Christ. Amen!

THIRD ROOT:

Traumas

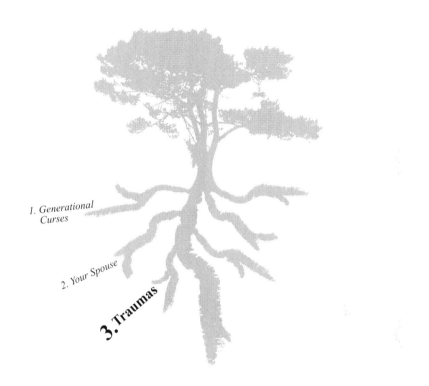

1. Generational Curses

2. Your Spouse

3. Traumas

We can see that some people develop a weight problem and/or hatred of their bodies following a traumatic experience. Each person reacts differently after an accident, the loss of a loved one, bankruptcy, sexual assault, etc.

Eating Our Emotions

Some people cannot manage their emotions, and they develop eating disorders. They start to "eat their emotions". By repeatedly eating without being hungry, we open a door to the enemy: the

> *By repeatedly eating without being hungry, we open a door to the enemy...*

devil. He will take great delight in providing you with all sorts of mental suggestions so you may yield to temptation.

There is a solution that will prevent us from falling into his trap. You must apologize to God for having discharged your emotions in food rather than have given Him these torments in prayer, for it is written:

> *"Let us walk honestly, as in the day; **not in rioting and drunkenness**, not in chambering and wantonness, not in strife and envying. But put ye on the Lord Jesus Christ, and make not provision for the flesh, to fulfil the lusts thereof."*
>
> *Romans 13:13-14*

Sexual Assault

However, for some people who have gone through a sexual assault, we see another possibility. They begin to gain weight afterwards, without having changed their eating habits. While they were slim before, they begin to gain weight.

> *"What? know ye not that he which is joined to an harlot is one body? for two, saith he, shall be one flesh."*
>
> *1 Corinthians 6:16*

You will notice that the person who caused the sexual abuse had a spirit of dependence and possibly weight issues. The Word of God says that when sex occurs between two people, they become "One" spiritually.

What was spiritually coming against the aggressor also came upon your life. If this is your case, reject this spirit in the name of Jesus Christ, as well as any spirit that came upon you through this sexual assault.

Say This Prayer:

Lord Jesus,

I thank you for the price you paid at the cross. You carried all my sufferings and all my pains.

The trauma I went through (name it: an accident, the loss of a loved one, bankruptcy, rejection...), I give it to you on this day. I apologize for having put my trust in food rather than in you, to eat when I was not hungry just to "feed" my pain, my dismay...

On this day, I give you the time(s) when I was sexually abused and I ask you to remove all emotional and psychological wounds that came upon me during this abuse.

I give you the anger and hatred I felt for that person. By your strength, I forgive him/her.

Now, in the powerful name of Jesus Christ, I take authority over every spirit that has spiritually come against me and I command them to immediately come out of my life, my soul, and my body.

I am washed by the blood of Jesus Christ, and free from the past.

In the name of Jesus Christ. Amen!

FOURTH ROOT:

Health Problems and Medication

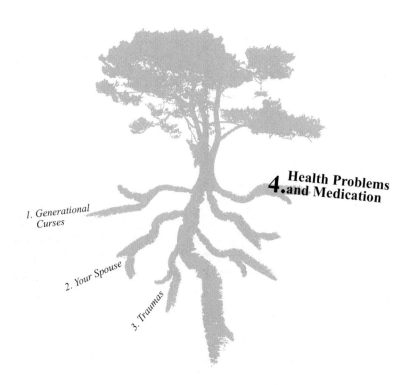

In this section, we will address health problems related to physical and/or psychological disorders, but also disorders pertaining to medication.

Medication

*M*any people, when they get sick, must take medication in the short, medium or long term. This medication may then influence their appetite and weight.

We can see that certain medications such as antidepressants, insulin and corticosteroids may contribute to weight gain and fat in the abdomen. These medications often cause a sense of hunger and therefore, they promote an increase in appetite. In the short, medium and long term, this has an impact on hormones, produces water retention in the body, alters blood flow, etc.

When hunger hits, ask the Holy Spirit: "Am I really hungry, or is it the effect of the medication?" Do not worry! The Lord will answer you! You know, people often do not dare to speak with the Lord, or do not think to pray to Him about the little things of everyday life. Yet, God finds pleasure in helping us and giving us victories in every detail of our lives, if we only ask Him...

> *God finds pleasure in helping us and giving us victories in every detail of our lives, if we only ask Him...*

Furthermore, by not committing sins of gluttony, we come into God's will. The more we are determined to do so, the more He will help us reach our goal. The Word of God says we must pray continually. You must be in unity with Him. It is good to pray alone in a room, on your knees, and in silence. However, prayer means talking to God, and we can get in a relationship with Him anytime, anywhere, and in all circumstances.

This is also why it is written that **when we are weak we are strong**. God is with us always. Certain situations are difficult? We could be weak, but we are not, because God is with us. His strength in us is stronger than the situation. Glory to God!

If you feel hungry for no reason, you should be aware that most of the time, the sensation of hunger is not real. It is triggered by the medication. By becoming aware that your stomach is not the one begging for food, you must resist and avoid eating at any time, and then you will overcome your false hunger.

> *His strength in us
> is stronger than the situation...*

Health Problems

Another important thing to understand is that physical health problems cause an individual to slow down his activities. This slowdown tends to make that person more sedentary and isolated. She is now tempted to eat more. All that is needed is to be aware of this habit and consciously refuse it.

Furthermore, medications can bring this slow down the person, causing her to feel more drained. So, you must proclaim victory in your physical health and refuse with authority to be overcome by the situation. I have seen so many people who were taking anti-depressants, begin to proclaim that they were healed. This was accomplished because the Lord renewed their strength. In the months that followed, they were completely healed and delivered! Hallelujah!

For others, we find that they have been medicated for some time and have gained weight. Even if they are no longer on medication, they kept the exceeding weight feeling uncomfortable because of it. It is therefore necessary for them to speak with authority and proclaim that their body gets back to its original shape before they had to start taking medications.

Say This Prayer:

Lord Jesus,

Forgive me for all the times I ate without being hungry.

Lord, I ask forgiveness for the sin of gluttony. I ask the Holy Spirit to teach me to discern the truth from the lie when I'm hungry or to show me when it's the medication that influences me.

Give me your strength Holy Spirit, to resist the temptation of eating for the wrong reasons.

Moreover, I ask you to remove the effects of the drug in my body, my blood and my hormones.

May all side effects, including weight gain, be immediately neutralized in the name of Jesus Christ.

Also, I receive what you paid for me at the cross, as it is written in Isaiah 53:5: "By His stripes I am healed."

In the name of Jesus Christ. Amen!

FIFTH ROOTH:

Ending Another Addiction

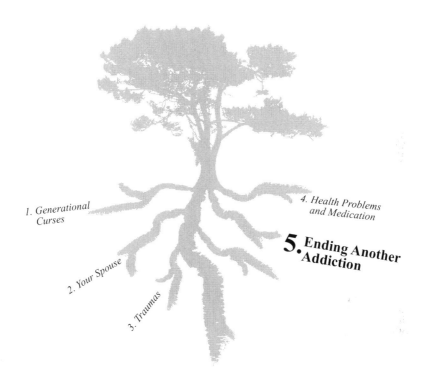

1. Generational Curses

4. Health Problems and Medication

5. Ending Another Addiction

2. Your Spouse

3. Traumas

I always noticed that people who were trying to remove something from their lives, without replacing it with something else, couldn't do it.

Generally, people who have developed an addiction of some kind (drugs, alcohol, emotional dependence, cigarettes, medication, etc.) engage in another type of dependence when they try to eliminate it from their lives. For example: someone who took cocaine will cease to use it, but will start smoking cigarettes and another one stops smoking, but begins eating more.

You certainly know people around you who are going through a painful time in their love life, and who "eat" their emotions. You understand the process... The person tried to remove the tree from their life by cutting down the trunk, but did not take the time to eliminate the problem at its root. After reading the teaching on the subject in this book, you now know that the problem is spiritual and not carnal. The person must deal with the root, which is a spirit of dependence.

Here are the weapons used by the spirit of addiction to destroy:

Dependence on alcohol, caffeine, cigarettes, drugs, food, medication, accusation, gluttony, hyperactivity, emotional dependency, compulsive behavior, perversion, condemnation, control, criticism, domination, submission, doubts about your Salvation, bashfulness, jealousy, insecurity, revenge, resentment, false compassion, false responsibility, fear of death, fear, frustration, nervousness, oppression, self-accusation, spiritual blindness, the need to feel superior, feeling lost, judging others, being possessive, condemnation of oneself.

Do you recognize a few of them that presently vex you? As you can see the spirit of dependence is the chief of "subordinate spirits". They manifest themselves in one form or another (gluttony, emotional dependence, etc.). You have within you the power to conquer them all. God has given you such power.

To help you better understand, imagine a (cruel) general that strategically puts his soldiers in place for you to lose the battle. The spirit of dependence is the general. To win the war, you must tackle the higher echelons instead of trying to fight the toy soldiers one by one. The "sub-spirits" will be automatically destroyed. You are part of the army of God and what is in you is stronger than anything that comes against you. **The army of God always comes out victorious of all battles when it perseveres. Our God is stronger than our adversary, and He lives in us.**

Take action against that spirit of dependence, or it will continue to be a harsh taskmaster if you do not face it.

> *You are part of the army of God and what is in you is stronger than anything that comes against you.*

Say This Prayer:

Lord Jesus,

You came on the cross to make me completely free. I gave you my life and through you, I am now free and liberated.

I ask your forgiveness for having been too dependent on food or on my image, rather than put my entire trust on you.

From this day on, I will be totally dependent on you. I shall not live by bread alone, but by every word coming out of the Word of God (Matthew 4:4).

Now, spirit of dependence, in the name of Jesus Christ, I command you to immediately come out of my life. You have no more power in my life.

I am dependent on God in every circumstance.

In the name of Jesus Christ. Amen!

SIXTH ROOT:

Fear

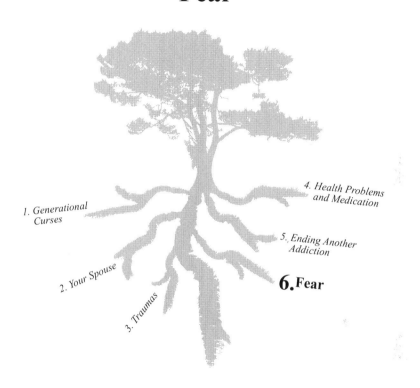

1. Generational Curses

2. Your Spouse

3. Traumas

4. Health Problems and Medication

5. Ending Another Addiction

6. Fear

nybody living in fear opens wide the door to Satan. He then comes in and affects them in the area corresponding to that fear in their lives.

Satan's kingdom works through fear, while the Kingdom of God operates by faith. Satan knows very well that if a human being accepts any type of fear, this means that he does not have faith in what the Word of God says and he can come in and play with that person's anxieties for as long as she lets him do it.

Satan's kingdom works through fear, while the Kingdom of God operates by faith.

Do not give him that pleasure! Take authority over the spirit of fear and throw it out in the name of Jesus Christ!

Fear:
The Ultimate Weapon of the Enemy

Fear does not come from God or from the Holy Spirit. It is written:

> *"For God hath not given us the spirit of fear; but of power, and of love, and of a sound mind."*
>
> *2 Timothy 1:7*

We have received the Holy Spirit, who is God's strength, His love and His wisdom.

*We have not received a **spirit of fear** but of power, love and **clarity of mind**.*

We have not received a **spirit of fear** but of power, love and **clarity of mind**. What a blessing!

98

As a child of God, we have not received a spirit of fear... So, if your fear is related to food, you must immediately reject this fear and counter it with the Word of God.

It is imperative to understand that we live under spiritual laws created by God and that these laws have an impact on every human being. Most people are familiar with this law: "Give and it shall be given you..." We see that business people who do well financially apply this spiritual principle. They are involved in charities, start a foundation, give to the poor, etc. And they receive even more in return!

What You Fear is What Afflicts You

We live, whether we like it or not, under the spiritual laws that God has created. One of these spiritual laws essential to understanding this chapter is the following: what you apprehend, or what you are afraid of (fear), is what afflicts you.

> *"**For the thing I greatly feared has come upon me, And what I dreaded has happened to me.** I am not at ease, nor am I quiet; I have no rest, for trouble comes."*
>
> *Job 3:25-26*

What I was Fearing was Happening to Me

It is interesting to see that what we fear, what we dread, is what attains us. In the Old Testament, Job opened the door to the adversary. The devil tormented him and won in the areas of his life where he was afraid of losing. I imagine that Job was not afraid of losing his wife, because she was not touched during the ordeal. She stayed with him until the end and gave him three more daughters, considered the three most beautiful women in the land…

This was a revelation for me, as far as my constant fear of gaining weight was concerned.

This was a revelation for me, as far as my constant fear of gaining weight was concerned. The adversary had the best part! I gave him all the power to torment me. Imagine that! I was replaying the story of Job. I was in a perpetual mode of failure and torment, totally clueless about what was happening to me.

This is the reason why you must eliminate all fears from your life and take authority over the dietary torment. Do not be fooled! Bind the thoughts that do not come from God and say: "On this day, I take captive my thoughts to make them obedient to Jesus Christ. Satan, I bind all thoughts of dietary torment coming from you. I reject them in the name of Jesus Christ. Amen!"

Do I Have Any Fears About Food and/or About My Body?

If you are among those who have trouble staying slim and are in constant struggle with food to maintain a slender body, clearly over the years you have bought into the enemy's fear tactics.

I had many fears related to food. Here are a few of them:

- Fear of eating chocolate... I would gain weight.
- Fear of eating bread, pasta or pastries... I was going to balloon up.
- Fear of gaining weight if I did not stay within the bounds of dietary restrictions.
- Fear of ever being slim for good and be free.
- Fear of being fat again, once my goal of thinness would be achieved.
- Fear... Fear... Fear...

You see, what I feared and dreaded the most actually happened in my life. Despite my best efforts in the natural, I was always returning to the same pattern. The will for getting out of it was not the problem.

I was imposing on myself all the restrictions, diets and exercises needed to achieve my goal, but I was subjected to the **spiritual laws of fear and faith**. I was inevitably attracting the results of my fears in my life. How many people have I seen in that same situation?

Year after year, diet after diet, this repetitive cycle turns your life into a true nightmare. The fears are becoming increasingly pervasive. **Today, when I look at these people, my heart writhes in pain within me.** I know they are subjected to the spiritual law of attraction and as long as they won't be aware of it and change their erroneous perception and programming, they will continue to experience the results of their fears year after year.

> *Year after year, diet after diet, this repetitive cycle turns your life into a true nightmare.*

Free and Slim People Are Not Afraid to Gain Weight!

Pause to reflect for a while. Think about the free and slim people that you know. They are not afraid of eating any one food in particular. The idea to gain weight does not even touch their spirit. Ask them! They won't hesitate to say they have no fear in this area of their lives. They will even often say: "Ah! I eat what I want and I never gain weight!"

Early in my relationship with Allen, I often told him I wanted to lose weight and I couldn't eat this or that. Each time, he replied: "Stop worrying about it! Eat what you like and if you're hungry, eat!"

102

Following Allen's Example

With time and the repetition of such a positive affirmation from him, I ultimately stopped being afraid of eating any type of food. **I watched Allen's attitude toward food and started to imitate him.** It is then, that from one day to the other, I became increasingly aware that fear was attracting exactly what I did not want... I refused it, as he did for himself.

Fear found a way into your mind also. Your emotions, or rather Satan played a nasty trick on you. This fear might have originated in your youth, when you heard family members talk about their fear of gaining weight. Did this fear begin while debating the subject with friends at school? Did this fear come while watching a newscast about the difficulty of losing weight after pregnancy or menopause? Did this fear appear after your doctor mentioned you could gain weight by taking such and such medication? At times, you felt the need to talk about your fear. You have a friend, the best! And his name is... **Jesus Christ! He is always listening to your desires and He answers them!**

Today, be aware of the fears you accepted in this area of your life. Make a list. Reject them and confess the Word of God through faith. You will be freed from your fear of chocolate, of not losing weight for good, etc.

> *"Therefore if the Son makes you free, you shall be free indeed."*
>
> *John 8:36*

Jesus Christ made you truly free: free from fear, any torment related to food and your body.

> *"The Spirit of the Sovereign LORD is on me, because the LORD has anointed me to preach good news to the poor. He has sent me to bind up the brokenhearted, **to proclaim freedom for the captives and release from darkness for the prisoners"***
>
> Isaiah 61:1 *(New International Version)*

The word "prisoners" in this verse comes from the Hebrew word "Acar", which means to be tied, bound, attacked, tormented and imprisoned by the adversary. Jesus Christ came to deliver, heal and set free all those who are tormented. By becoming a child of God through Jesus Christ, you are delivered from all torments and fear by His blood, shed on the cross, and you are released... Released in your thoughts, your emotions, and your body. Hallelujah!

Today, be aware of the fears
you accepted in this area of your life...
And reject them!

Say This Prayer:

Lord Jesus,

Thank you for sending me the Holy Spirit, who is not a spirit of fear or of timidity, but a spirit of strength, power, love, and wisdom. I now walk by faith and not by fear.

I trust in what your Word says about me and not in thoughts of fear that came to my life through the years. I believe for the best, for my body and myself.

I do not fear what the world fears about their body, food and old age.

The closer I get to you, the more beautiful I get, and the more I reflect your glory.

I take authority over all the fears I accepted in the past (name the fears regarding food and your weight) and I reject them from my life.

In the name of Jesus Christ. Amen!

7. SEVENTH ROOT:

The Root Of All Roots:
Gluttony

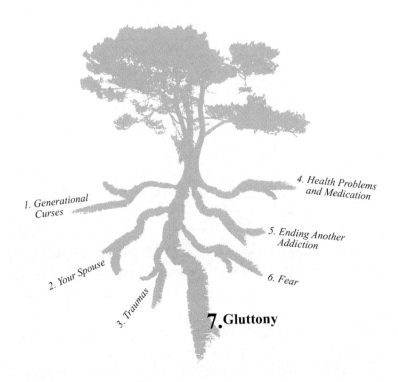

1. Generational Curses

4. Health Problems and Medication

5. Ending Another Addiction

2. Your Spouse

6. Fear

3. Traumas

7.Gluttony

his chapter addresses for each and all the deepest root, which is the foundation of all others. This root must be absolutely burnt to a crisp and immediately eliminated from your life if you want the 7 keys to be effective and ensure your absolute victory.

A spiritual foundation has settled in your life to create this problem of overeating. Whether it be generational curses, traumas, spouse issues, health problems, ending another addiction or fear.

Gluttony Is A Sin

This foundation, this root has been established by a sin of overeating generated either by you or by previous generations. The sin has been gluttony, overeating. The only way Satan uses to make havoc in a person's life and gain a specific territory is when a human opens him the door, accepts him in his life and yields to temptation. Be aware of it! **You have more power than you think.**

Few people realize that gluttony is a sin. Many make jokes about it, openly and consciously sinning. However, these same people (as a child of God) know that fornication, magic and greed are sins, but they make abstraction of gluttony as being one!

Few people realize that gluttony is a sin.

Yet the same verse tells us overeating is a sin.

*"Now the works of the flesh are manifest, which are these; Adultery, **fornication**, uncleanness, lasciviousness, idolatry, **witchcraft**, hatred, variance, emulations, wrath, strife, seditions, heresies, envyings, murders, drunkenness, **revellings**, and such like: of the which I tell you before, as I have also told you in time past, that they which do such things shall not inherit the kingdom of God."*
                                     Galatians 5:19-21

As you can see, "revellings" (overeating, also translated as "orgies" in the NIV and NASB versions of the Bible) are part of the same list as fornication, magic and envy. They are as reprehensible as the other sins... Did you know this? If not, it's time to revise your way of thinking...

Warning! I desire to inform you that this truth is not accusatory, but I mentioned it so you would understand that this sin, when sustained, opens a door to the enemy. It can easily destroy you in this area of your life. Never forget that the tempter is the devil and his basic strategy is to entice you. Remember the story of Jesus in the desert... (*Matthew 4:1-4*).

By making you succumb to temptation and sin, the enemy gives himself an entry to continue his destructive work. There is no shortage of tricks in his bag since he is the master of deception. He will enter through the smallest door, for example, with a thought of gluttony that will cross your mind. Do not give him control over you in any way. Just stop being influenced so easily, especially if you know that behind this thought there is a demon that pushes you to act. The time has come to reclaim your rights! As a child of God, put on the full armor of God, be strong in the Lord by rereading, praying and meditating on *Ephesians 6:10-18* :

> *"Finally, my brethren, be strong in the Lord, and in the power of his might. **Put on the whole armour of God, that ye may be able to stand against the wiles of the devil. For we wrestle not against flesh and blood, but against principalities, against powers, against the rulers of the darkness of this world, against spiritual wickedness in high places**. Wherefore take unto you the whole armour of God, that ye may be able to withstand in the evil day, and having done all, to stand. **Stand therefore**, having your loins girt about with truth, and having on the breastplate of righteousness; And your feet shod with the preparation of the gospel of peace; Above all, taking the shield of faith, wherewith ye shall be able to quench all the fiery darts of the wicked. And take the helmet of salvation, and the sword of the Spirit, which is the word of God: Praying always with all prayer and supplication in the Spirit, and watching thereunto with all perseverance and supplication for all saints."*

With generational curses, the sin of gluttony found its roots in your bloodline, and you have unavoidably inherited it. As we already realized in previous roots, it's so easy to commit the sin of gluttony.

If, after a trauma, you released your emotions by eating when you were not hungry, and kept it up, this sin of gluttony built its foundation. If it's because you've had sexual inter-course with someone who was overweight and/or had an eating disorder, this sin had an impact in your life. If it's because you ate more as a side effect of drugs without necessarily being hungry, you've opened a door to the enemy. If you ate for two while pregnant, you were gluttonous, etc.

*"All things are lawful unto me, but all things are not expedient: all things are lawful for me, but **I will not be brought under the power of any. Meats for the belly, and the belly for meats:** but God shall destroy both it and them. **Now the body is not for fornication**, but for the Lord; and the Lord for the body."*

1 Corinthians 6:12-13

I will not let myself be enslaved by anything... I am not enslaved by food. Food is not my dependence, it's only for my belly and that's it! It's not for my emotions, and I'm not controlled by food.

"For of whom a man is overcome, of the same is he brought in bondage."

2 Peter 2:19b

Reject the temptations of the devil in your life. The sin of gluttony and the devil's attractive suggestions or mental insinuations abound. He hisses words like: "You have not eaten enough. Look how too thin you are because of all your deprivation, etc." He finds all the places and circumstances to make you fall and reach his objective.

> *Food is not my dependence, it's only for my belly and that's it! It's not for my emotions, and I'm not controlled by food.*

If Satan knows your weakness is food, he will put people and objects of covetousness that will obviously be difficult to resist. He will use confusing emotional situations to get you to eat more. Once dependence is well established, all he needs to do is whisper a few thoughts in your mind from time to time to keep this sin going.

Reject it altogether! Even if he seems very strong, you are more powerful than he by the power God has given you. Stop being a slave to food! Cherish your freedom in Jesus Christ. **You must take care of your body, which is the temple of the Holy Spirit.**

*"Know ye not that ye are the temple of God, and that the Spirit of God dwelleth in you? If any man defile the temple of God, him shall God destroy; for **the temple of God is holy, which temple ye are.**"*

1 Corinthians 3.16-17

You are holy and must remain holy. Do not think a little overeating at a special occasion is not a serious matter. Could I ask if it's acceptable for you to kiss your friend's husband or wife only once at a dinner party because he/she is an irresistible beauty? Would it be normal to hear people say: "I have kissed or had sex with my brother's wife at Christmas because she smelled so nice! It was a special occasion and I couldn't resist!"

In the list where sexual immorality (fornication) and uncleanness are mentioned, we also find overeating! It is as unacceptable to overeat during special occasions (weddings, Christmas, vacations...) than to kiss your sister's husband! You must always resist this temptation! I did say always! In God's sight, it's the same sin, as surprising as it may seem. You will certainly see things differently now that you're aware of it as a child of God. It is written that God's people perish for lack of knowledge *(Hosea 4:6)*. If you are constantly struggling with food, switching between moments of deprivation and excess, it is time to readjust your way of thinking. These two extremes are in disagreement with God's will for you.

The Sin of Gluttony Was In My Bloodline

When I was young, the sin of gluttony was in my bloodline. Since nobody had broken it in the name of Jesus Christ, of course I inherited it in my life. I was not eating excessively, but fears conveyed in the conversations during meals began permeate my soul. I grew up and started gaining weight around the age of 12. All my fears showed up at that time. I was so afraid to have a body like the women in my family that it happened! You already know the rest of my story...

> *I was not eating excessively, but fears conveyed in the conversations during meals began permeate my soul.*

I especially want to bring your attention to the **main problem, which was that the previous generational sin had not been broken in my life. This curse was unfairly making me gain weight. Problem number two is not hard to imagine: in turn, I repeated the sin of gluttony and deprivation**. And this is the pattern passed on from one generation to the next. But glory to God, this is broken for good! Future generations will not have to suffer from it!

You must make a firm decision to reject this sin in your life. No matter if it came through one or more of the aforementioned roots, the most important thing is to repent of this sin today. Take authority over that spirit of dependence in the name of Jesus Christ and remove it from your life!

"And the prayer of faith shall save the sick, and the Lord shall raise him up; and if he have committed sins, they shall be forgiven him. Confess your faults one to another, and pray one for another, that ye may be healed. The effectual fervent prayer of a righteous man availeth much."

James 5:15-16

Confess this sin and you'll be healed,
healed from torments and
healed in your body.

Hallelujah!

By steering clear of **overeating,** you will be able to:

- Prevent the enemy from having power over your body.

- Stop feeling bad and bloated.

- Remove any territory to the spirit of dependence. It will be impossible for him to play with your appetite, your body and your hormones.

- Prevent the enemy's thoughts (accusations, guilt...) from tormenting you.

Say This Prayer:

Heavenly Father,

I come before you now in the name of Jesus Christ. I repent from the sins of gluttony, deprivation and not loving myself on several occasions. I repent from all conscious or unconscious sins I committed.

I'm sorry for anything that displeased you or anything that could have separated me from you. Wash me with your blood, wash me and fill me with the Holy Spirit in the name of Jesus Christ.

I bring my thoughts captive in you today. My thoughts are bounded with your thoughts, my will to your will. I bind my feet in the path of righteousness, and walk according to your will, in the name of Jesus Christ.

I command to be loosed from any path outside of your will, thoughts and actions that are not from you. Thank you for delivering me, and I thank you Lord for this day of victory and progress.

I ask you to show me in advance all of Satan's plans, tactics, and strategies against me today. I come against, I stop and forsake any bad emotion bound to my soul, every curse spoken or written or expressed in any way against me in this day.

I speak forgiveness and loose my entire lineage from past generations who have sinned and put curses in my bloodline.

I break the power of any curse caused by the sins of glutonny, hatred, and dependence that have come from my bloodline or me. I break the power of any curse that came through my bloodline: witchcraft, astral projections, Satanism, spiritualism, psychic practices, Indian curses, voodooist, Santeria, or of any other curse spoken through my bloodline.

I reverse this curse and send those demons back where they came from in the name of Jesus Christ. Father, in the name of Jesus Christ, I have repented and I now repent from the sin of gluttony.

I have confessed and I now confess this sin of food abuse and ask you to forgive me.

I take authority over every foul spirit that came into my life through this sin, and I take authority over every spirit that came because of this sin, such as diabetes, hypoglycemia or other diseases.

I command you to leave me immediately in the name of Jesus Christ. On this day Lord, I decide to turn to you.

On every occasion, I will turn to you and not to food. From now on you will be my source and I give you my anxieties, stress and emotions.

Now Satan, I command you, and your kingdom, to leave in the name of Jesus Christ. I chose Jesus Christ as my Lord and Savior, and on this day Satan, I renounce all your temptations.

Lord, I thank you for everything you have done for me, your child, because I believed in your name. Thank you Lord for becoming a curse on the cross to redeem me from all curses.

In the name of Jesus Christ. Amen!

Section Three

THE 777 PROGRAM

7Keys For an Absolute Victory
7Minutes Per Day
7Weeks

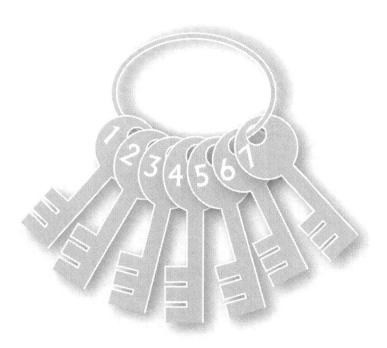

First Week
1ˢᵗ Key:

The Power of Decision

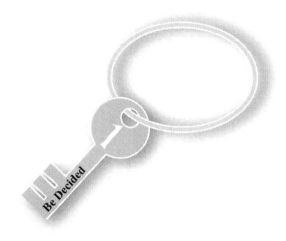

"A single decision will affect your destiny."

THE POWER OF DECISION

his first key is the essential foundation for the success of the six other keys. By taking hold of all keys, your soul will be powerfully "muscled" and the enemy will not be able to keep you captive in this pattern that prevented you from living the true life in Jesus Christ. Glory to God for his powerful Word! Now, you must be determined. It is the secret of this first key to find or regain your freedom and your slenderness. The power of it will inevitably propel you toward an absolute victory. **It is the engine of the process of success.**

At this stage of your reading, you are in a position to decide if you want to tackle the right root of the problem head on or return to your previous programming. It's your choice. You can decide to think like most people do or as God teaches us to do. You can decide to keep the problem in your life and not deal with it or to get rid of it once and for all!

> *You may choose to think like most people do or as God teaches us to do.*

Remember that you can't conquer what you don't confront and you can't confront what you have not identified. Since we have found the root of the problem in the second chapter, you are now able to confront the right problem and conquer it.

You understand that the root of all roots is spiritual and that it's located in your soul. It now becomes your choice, your decision to deal with it properly and be completely victorious.

Choice, Not Chance Determines Our Destiny

As long as we tolerate a situation, we don't apply the necessary effort to change it. **Act like a winner! Be a person of conviction!** Do you want to see this situation change in your life? You must want it badly and make it your priority. It is of first importance to uphold your decision and stick to it. If this is not important for you or if you take this too lightly, it won't work. The enemy (the devil) can make you spin around in circles so you don't know which way to turn anymore. He enjoys confusing you... He buys time playing with your mind. He does it to win! As he puts doubts and confusion in your head, he moves strategically. Keep your eyes on the goal. Keep going forward, despite the obstacles. If you fall... Pick yourself up!

Keep your eyes on the goal. Keep going forward, despite the obstacles. If you fall... Pick yourself up!

It's now critical to be a soldier of God who marches with the desire to feel good about himself. Be rigorous in order to "muscle" your soul and offer a total resistance to the devil so he can definitely flee!

Show good will and keep your eyes fixed on the Word of God, and not on human wisdom. As the Word of God says: "The wisdom of man is foolishness to God and God's wisdom is foolishness to man." *(1 Cor. 1:25, 1 Cor. 3:19)* This day, choose God's wisdom and you will see that our God is good.

> *To get different results,*
> *we must be prepared to act differently.*

With This Key:

- **Be determined** to face the real root of the problem.

- **Be determined** to put on the whole armor of God.

- **Be determined** to receive and apply the Word of God in this area of your life.

- **Be determined** to get your victory.

- **Be determined** to take your victory.

- **Be determined** to go and get this blessing.

- **Be determined** to be once and for all at peace in your head.

- **Be determined** to be once and for all at peace in your emotions regarding your body and food.

- **Be determined** not to exceed the limits of your appetite.

- **Be determined** to tell this spirit you have victory over him.

- **Be decided** to tell this spirit that you are slim.

- **Be determined** to starve this spirit, and see yourself totally delivered and feel it.

- **Be determined** to renew your mind and be deprogrammed from the manner by which this spirit keeps you captive.

- **Be determined** to have absolute victory in this area of your life.

- **Be determined** to resist gluttony.

- **Be determined** to no longer deprive yourself of food as a way of losing weight.

By being determined, you will see your life completely transformed. By being determined, your thoughts will change. You will feed on the truth, you will begin to think differently and have different results. **Repeating the "Be determined" motto is voluntary on my part, because it is the secret of the first key, so essential that it comes before all other ones.** Take the time to assimilate this teaching before going forward. Meditate on every sentence to permeate yourself with them. Your success depends on it!

Being definitely determined is an important success factor... I know it! However, you should know that you're undertaking a battle: **You are deciding to get up and face an adversary who occupied territory for too long in your life already. Know that this fight requires being rigorous and to always keep your eyes on the result.**

> *Being determined is an important success factor...*
> *I know it!*

Be a Boxer

When a boxer gets in the ring, he has one goal in mind, the end result... And the result is winning. Do you have the same objective as the boxer? He knows that the fight will require energy, endurance and that if he falls to the mat, he will recover and continue till the victory. He has only one thing in mind: bringing down the opponent to the mat. He doesn't doubt and you must duplicate this example in your life. **He's not on the defensive, but the offensive, and this makes all the difference.** You must do the same thing. Ignore the enemy's attacks or wiles, but hang onto your victory with all your might. Some attacks may come from your relatives. Here are some possible reactions from you family: "You do not eat more? Have you become anorexic? Are you sick? You're not as beautiful when you're slim." Don't let yourself be influenced... It's your decision and not that of others!

You must now choose to believe the Word of God and not the lies the enemy will try to whisper in your ear. Remember that the goal of this process is to obtain an absolute victory for your freedom and your slenderness. **This is not another weight loss method or some new psychoanalysis of your past to free yourself... This is the truth of God applied in this area of your life, that will release your true physical destiny and perfect body that God has for you.**

Say This Prayer:

On this day Lord, I decide to forego the temptation to eat with gluttony. I renounce the temptation to overeat or to deprive myself when I'm hungry in the name of Jesus Christ.

I render my thoughts captive in you Lord; my thoughts are bound to your thoughts, my will to your will.

I bind my feet in the path of righteousness and walk according to your will. I will eat only when I'm hungry and stop eating when I'm not hungry anymore.

Today, I have decided to win. I decide to receive and live the abundant life that Jesus Christ paid for me. On this day, I decide to deny and invalidate any negative thought, every lie of the enemy. I decide to feed on the Word of God, of your truth Lord.

Today, I declare and decree over my life that I am free and delivered from every torment regarding food. I am delivered from every torment against my body.

I declare and decree that I feel good in my skin. I feel good in my thoughts. I feel good in my emotions and in my body.

Lord, I declare that I am blessed coming in, and blessed going out. Everything my hands touch is blessed. I have life and life in abundance, because I now follow you Lord, and do not walk in darkness anymore.

I hear your voice. I choose you. I choose to obey, obey your voice on this day, in the name of Jesus Christ.

Body, I command you in the name of Jesus Christ: you are immediately and supernaturally restored and recreated to the original shape God intended, which is to say, perfect.

In the name of Jesus Christ. Amen!

Applying the Principles

- Take time to understand the previous lessons to obtain a complete divine victory.

- Be determined to face the root(s) of the problem you have identified in the second chapter. This is important!

- Close the door to all your fears in the name of Jesus Christ. No demon can stop you if you are determined.

- Be determined to take authority over what comes against you and to reprogram yourself according to the Word of God.

- Do not deprive yourself. Frustration and deprivation are not from God.

- Be determined to become slim and you will. Think differently, and it will be accomplished in the name of Jesus Christ!

- Everyday, over the next seven weeks, read again the "Be determined…" list.

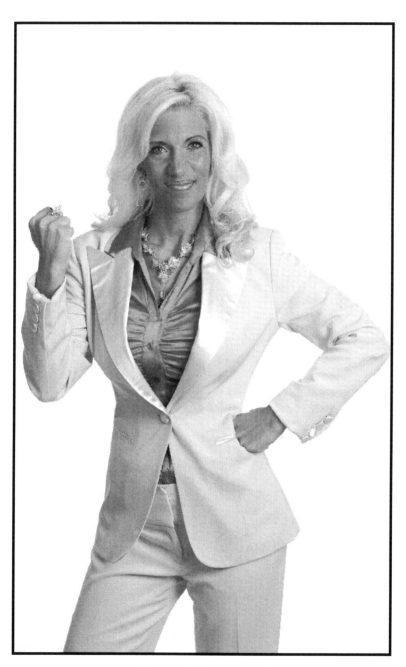

Be a Boxer!

SECOND WEEK

2ND KEY:

DEPROGRAMMING "VIRUSES" AND REPROGRAMMING ACCORDING TO THE WORD OF GOD

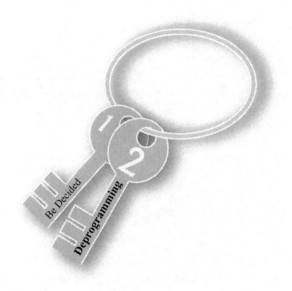

"God wants to renew your life by renewing your mind."

DEPROGRAMMING VIRUSES AND REPROGRAMMING ACCORDING TO THE WORD OF GOD

his key is so precious! When we get hold of it and understand this revelation, **all that was impossible to man becomes possible with God's truth.**

Understand that when you became a child of God, you became a NEW CREATION! As a new creation, you don't think like the old one. You are not the same. You no longer act the same way.

Are you a child of God? If so, then you must think like the Word of God tells you to. You do not think like people in the world. You think as your heavenly Father thinks. Remember that God's wisdom is foolishness to man. You cannot simply read the Bible without applying its principles.

> *"But be ye doers of the word, and not hearers only, deceiving your own selves. For if any be a hearer of the word, and not a doer, he is like unto a man beholding his natural face in a glass: For he beholdeth himself, and goeth his way, and straightway forgetteth what manner of man he was. But whoso looketh into the perfect law of liberty, and continueth therein, he being not a forgetful hearer, but a doer of the work, this man shall be blessed in his deed."*
>
> *James 1:22-25*

These teachings will strengthen you as you go deeper into them, and they will transform the inner workings of your mind. The Word of God is a river of living water that fills you and cleanses you, which transforms your current programming pattern. If you're unfamiliar with the Bible, start with the verses that you find throughout this book.

This second key consists in telling you what you need to deprogram within yourself. "Viruses" (lies of the devil) have been "injected" into your mind. The second key will allow you to reprogram yourself with the truth of the Word of God. Believe me... It works, because the Word of God does not return void!

> *"So shall my word be that goeth forth out of my mouth: it shall not return unto me void, but it shall accomplish that which I please, and it shall prosper in the thing whereto I sent it."*
> *Isaiah 55:11*

Switching From the World's System to God's System

"And be not conformed to this world: but be ye transformed by the renewing of your mind, that ye may prove what is that good, and acceptable, and perfect, will of God."

Romans 12:2

If I want to be transformed, I must renew my mind by the Word of God.

This verse is so powerful and revealing! **For years, I thought like the world and got the same results as the world, despite the fact that I was a Christian.** This verse is clear. If I want to be transformed, I must renew my mind by the Word of God. Because God created me perfect and slim, I must return to the source: Jesus Christ. I have been remodeled to the original shape God had given me, and not based on what Satan wanted to do with me.

I grew up with lies, thoughts contrary to God's mind. These seeds had a negative impact on my self-esteem, my relationship with food and my body. **I have named these lies viruses.** They prevented me from living a normal life long enough.

Viruses In Your Life

It's like a computer that gets infected with viruses. When viruses get into a computer, they prevent it from performing to its full capacity, maybe even cause a significant deficiency, or worse yet, shut it down altogether. If you want to restore it to its proper operation, you must identify and remove the viruses, and sometimes reprogram specific databases that have been disrupted by them.

Regarding this area of your life, it is certain that you have received "viruses" in your soul that affected your relationship with food and by extension, your slenderness. Now, you must consciously remove them from your mind and subsequently, reprogram yourself with the truth of the Word of God, which becomes your "antivirus".

> *When viruses get into a computer, they prevent it from performing to its full capacity, maybe even cause a significant deficiency, or worse yet, shut it down altogether.*

The world's way of thinking about our perception of weight and how to eat is not God's way. Firstly, we see through statistics that people who diet fail 95% of the time. It's clear that diets don't work and besides, God does not want us to be in any kind of food restrictions, or fear, anxiety and deprivation. Jesus Christ came to give us abundant life and for me, abundance includes the joy of eating what you love. Don't rob me of the joy of eating a delicious cheesecake! This is part of my abundance! I'm entitled to it! **However, God doesn't want me to be dependent on the cheesecake. I must not abuse it. I hope I make myself clear on this particular point.**

> *Don't rob me of the joy of eating a delicious cheesecake! This is part of my abundance!*

"for of whom a man is overcome, of the same is he brought in bondage."

2 Peter 2:19b

The War Zone: Your Soul

Paul the Apostle mentions in Romans 12:2 that we are transformed by the renewing of our minds. The battle is in our thoughts and our intelligence; it is precisely there that you must have victory.

It is proven that 85% of everything a human being does is connected to the programming of his subconscious mind. What you think and say, as well as how you act toward food and your body is 85% programmed since your childhood. Everyday, you repeat the same negative thoughts and attitudes. What's happening?

Day after day, you get the same unfavorable results, the same patterns that are so harmful to your well-being and fulfillment. But today, while reading these lines, give glory to

God, for your thoughts and attitudes will be deprogrammed from the enemy's lies and reprogrammed with the truth.

Observe **free** and **slim** people around you. You can **see** their programming regarding food and their body is not at all the same as yours. **Whatever the root that brought this problem in your life, this root will not be able to resist the truth and its application in your life.**

When my life radically changed after devoting myself to the Lord, I realized how the Bible was such a contemporary book, and an essential practical tool to gain victory in every detail of my daily life. This book is so wonderful! Thank you Lord for your unparalleled love toward us, and your Word that frees us! Thank you Lord!

You Become What You Think

From this chapter on, your mindset will change, so that the results will be noticeable. I call this the start of your soul's muscular training. Now we remove the "viruses" that you've accepted from your childhood. We will then work to reprogram your mind. Free and slim people see themselves as being slender; they have no fear of gaining weight. It's impossible for them to be overweight. What they think is what they are.

In fact, we become what we think throughout the day. A human being has an average of 60,000 thoughts per day and

A human being has an average of 60,000 thoughts per day and 90% of these thoughts are repetitive.

90% of these thoughts are repetitive. The more you reprogram your mind with the truth through repetition, the more these truths will grow roots deep within your intellect. What is important to note is that a negative thought can be repeated up to 600 times a day. Imagine then the impact of a lie from the enemy against your body and/or food that is repeated over 600 times in one day... Imagine two or ten negative thoughts and more... You understand that it is time for you to think differently and program yourself correctly.

This is why it's important to immediately get rid of all negative thoughts you may entertain: any thought that disagree with the Word of God and all of the enemy's lies. Replace them with the truth, which is the Word of God.

Here are some of the lies that free people and slim people do not believe:

- If I eat this or that (cake, pasta, chips...), I'll put on weight.
- If I continue eating (while still being hungry; remember that free and slim people don't eat when they're no longer hungry), I'll gain weight.

- If I don't have lunch, I'll be sick.
- It's imperative that I take three meals a day and two snacks.
- It's noon, I have to eat.
- I have to finish my plate.
- It's not polite to leave food on my plate.
- If I go to a restaurant, I have to get my money's worth and more, especially at a buffet.
- I have to count calories so I don't gain weight.
- I ate more than 1,200 calories during the day, I will surely gain weight.
- Anything makes me gain weight.
- It's normal to gain weight at menopause.
- It's so difficult to lose weight after pregnancy.
- Etc.

You can see that these are lies, "viruses" transmitted by those who are not free in this area of their lives. They are not free with food. Free and slim people don't believe these lies. Now you need to start thinking and seeing yourself the way slim and free people do, if you want the same results. Free yourself from all these false statements from the people in the world!

Your Prevalent Attitude:
Live in Freedom and Slenderness

You must keep your eyes open on what you want and not on what you don't want. Adopt a new attitude: see yourself free and slim right now! Focus your attention on the fact

Adopt a new attitude:
see yourself free and slim
right now!

that you already have your victory and that obviously, it's already done. Think like a slim person to become... slim yourself!

"Therefore I tell you, whatever you ask for in prayer, believe that you have received it, and it will be yours."

Mark 11:24

Reprogram yourself now by way of the inner workings of free and slim people. Here are some examples of questions to be programmed in your mind so you don't fall in the enemy's trap.

Do you:

- Eat out of habit, or because you're really hungry?
- Usually eat breakfast or are you really hungry?
- Eat three meals a day as a tradition or are you really hungry?
- Act like a glutton because of the smell (it smells so good!), the beauty (it looks so beautiful and good!), or do you really want to eat the food?
- Eat out of boredom, loneliness, sadness, anger... Or are you really hungry?
- Snack out of habit, boredom, or are you really hungry?

When you feel like you're still hungry just after finishing up your meal, ask yourself:

- Is it because I have not had enough to eat?
- Is it because I'm thirsty?
- Is it because I'm tired?
- Is it because I'm angry? ...I feel alone? ...I feel neglected and/or abandoned? ...I'm stressed? ... I'm worried?

Here's what free and slim people think and do, and what you must do in return:

- Do not stay away from foods you love. You'll end up craving too much for them.
- You were created with personal preferences. Do not ignore who you are. Accept who you are and what you like will accept you...
- Do not deprive yourself. Deprivation and frustration are the sworn enemies of slenderness.
- When you no longer want to eat, but there's still food in your plate, I like to deposit my napkin or my utensils in the plate. Or you can simply get rid of it.
- Drink between meals.
- Do not feel guilty when, on certain days, you have more appetite. This is normal... All free and slim people eat more on certain days.
- Do not force yourself to eat if you're not hungry. Some days are like that... All free and slim people eat less on certain days.

144

Think and Act As Those Who Have No "Virus"

Day after day, you have to deprogram your mind from these lies that stop your freedom and your slenderness. **These "viruses" are "blockers".** You can counter them by becoming aware of your mental programming toward food and your body, then by modifying it as we've seen previously.

Eventually, you will change your destiny. God wants you to think as He thinks, and as a person who doesn't have any "virus" in this area of his or her life.

Understand that God created things this way. You must have your thoughts on what you want, not on what you do not want. The apostle Paul had his thoughts fixed on his ultimate goal: to go to Rome to meet with Cae-

> *Day after day, you have to deprogram your mind from these lies that stop your freedom and your slenderness. These "viruses" are "blockers".*

sar and bring the Good News of the Kingdom of God to the pagans. He was not alone. When we look at Scriptures, we see several stories of men and women of God who kept their eyes on what they wanted and were victorious. Here are a few examples: Nehemiah with the walls of Jerusalem, Moses with Pharaoh, Joshua with Jericho, Naomi with Ruth and Boaz, etc. All these people have focused their attention on the desired result, and not on the prevailing circumstances. Do the same!

Your Mental Image

> *If you believe that food has control over your body, well, it will be so, and you'll always be a slave.*

Following in their footsteps, generate the desired and necessary changes in your life. You have the power! From now on, see yourself as being slim so that it becomes a reality. You must feel free in your relationship with food to be really free. If you believe that food has control over your body, well, it will be so, and you'll always be a slave.

You must now reject all the thoughts that have been programmed by this spirit that came against you. He programmed you to accept all sorts of lies that free and slim people do not believe. If you want to be like these people, make sure you think the same way.

You could tell me it's not logical, but remember that God's wisdom is foolishness to man, and the spiritual laws God created are irreversible. God says that what you believe is what you receive.

> *"And Jesus said unto the centurion, Go thy way; and as thou hast believed, so be it done unto thee. And his servant was healed in the selfsame hour."*
>
> *Matthew 8:13*

Today and forever, you must always be offensive and you'll begin to think and act as a free and slim person.

> *"Therefore I say unto you, What things soever ye desire, when ye pray, believe that ye receive them, and ye shall have them."*
>
> Mark 11:24

Take Hold of Your Victory

Believe it's already done! Seize your victory now! Do not rely on the present circumstances and do not cling to the past. Keep your eyes on your victory and act as though it was already done, because you BELIEVE you already received it. Hallelujah!

It is critically important that you understand that your absolute success with this key will only come if you apply its principles day after day, minute by minute. Each of your thoughts will have an impact on your victory. **You can't get rich by thinking and acting like a poor person.** It's exactly the same thing for this type of victory in your life!

The greatest athletes and successful people will tell you they always see their success before it becomes a reality in their lives.

147

You can't be free and slim by thinking and acting like someone that's enslaved to food and by seeing yourself as obese.

The greatest athletes and successful people will tell you they always see their success before it becomes a reality in their lives. From now on, you must see your success as a reality.

> "*But let him ask in faith, nothing wavering. For **he that wavereth** is like a wave of the sea driven with the wind and tossed. For **let not that man think that he shall receive any thing of the Lord. A double minded man is unstable in all his ways.**"*
>
> *James 1:6-8*

Eliminate Doubt

Your doubts, as well as all your negative thoughts and emotions, are at odds with the Word and the will of God for your life. It's not your thoughts and emotions that control you! Do not let the enemy invade your mind and manipulate you with his lying and conniving thoughts that impose a weight on your faith and your emotions. You are stronger than the enemy.

> *You are stronger than the enemy. What is in you is stronger than what comes against you.*

148

What is in you is stronger than what comes against you.
Jesus Christ triumphed over the enemy over 2,000 years ago!
You received the Holy Spirit, the same spirt who raised Jesus
Christ from the dead. He lives in you, and everything that is
born of God overcomes the world. Glory to God!

> *"But if the Spirit of him that raised up Jesus
> from the dead dwell in you, he that raised up
> Christ from the dead shall also quicken your
> mortal bodies by his Spirit that dwelleth in
> you."*
>
> *Romans 8:11*

> *"For whatsoever is born of God overcometh the
> world: and this is the victory that overcometh
> the world, even our faith."*
>
> *1 John 5:4*

Say This Prayer:

Welcome Holy Spirit.

Fill this entire space today.

Thank you Lord, because my body is yours and my thoughts are your thoughts. I am slimmer and slimmer. I feel free. I am free in my relationship with food. I feel better and better in my body.

You are with me, and you protect my thoughts. You want success for me and I feel good. I feel good in my body.

Victory is mine! I'm ready for battle, and I'm successful.

*I praise you Lord. I am fearfully and wonderfully made, a marvelous creation indeed. I praise you Lord, because I am **a marvelous creation!** I praise you Lord, because **I am a marvelous creation!!!** **Hallelujah!***

I'm wonderful! Everything I touch succeeds!

In the name of Jesus Christ. Amen!

Applying the Principles

- You have become a new creature in Jesus Christ. Think like a new creature of God.

- Eliminate immediately all thoughts about your body and food, which are contrary to the will of God.

- Diets and dietary restrictions are no longer part of your life.

- Confess the truth of the Word of God over your body and in connection with your total deliverance from food.

- You now see yourself as being free and slim.

- You focus on what you want and not on what you do not want.

- Do not look at the state of your body, but rather look at the state of your thoughts that will change your body.

- Be proactive as soon as you wake up in the morning and glorify God for this miracle in your life.

- Even if on some days you don't feel good about yourself, refuse and reject that emotion and that thought in the name of Jesus Christ, and repeat out loud that you feel good in your skin, you are slim and you're a marvelous creation.

- Keep this book within reach everyday 7 days a week for the next 7 weeks. Read and reread it. Your mind needs to be reprogrammed with the truth of God.

- Stop nibbling out of habit, to pass the time, out of boredom, or to have something in your mouth. Eat only when you're hungry.

THIRD WEEK

3ᴿᴰ KEY:

UNDERSTANDING AND USING OUR AUTHORITY AS A CHILD OF GOD

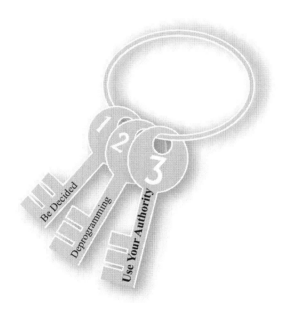

"Your life is a boat, and you're the captain."

UNDERSTANDING AND USING OUR AUTHORITY AS A CHILD OF GOD

his key will allow you to understand, receive, and release this authority, the power of God that is in you, to get your total deliverance and achieve your slenderness. The Word of God says that Jesus Christ delivered us from the power of darkness (*Colossians 1:13*), He redeemed us from the curse (*Galatians 3:13*) and he has given us **the authority** to defeat the enemy:

> *"Behold, I give unto you power to tread on serpents and scorpions, and over all the power of the enemy: and nothing shall by any means hurt you."*
>
> *Luke 10:19*

> *"But ye shall receive power, after that the Holy Ghost is come upon you: and ye shall be witnesses unto me both in Jerusalem, and in all Judaea, and in Samaria, and unto the uttermost part of the earth."*
>
> *Acts 1:8*

As you read earlier, The root of the root of the problem is spiritual, and you have no other choice but to attack this root. To confront it head on, you must take hold of the spiritual weapons.

154

"For though we walk in the flesh, we do not war after the flesh. **For the weapons of our warfare are not carnal**, *but mighty through God to the pulling down of strong holds."*

2 Corinthians 10:3-4

The Spirit That Raised Jesus Christ From the Dead Lives In You

You do not fight according to the flesh. To eliminate this problem once and for all, it's necessary to burn the roots. This key is exactly one of the extremely effective spiritual weapons for reversing all the fortresses that came against you. You must realize that you received supernatural strength when you became a child of God. Few Christians realize this, and it is really time that God's people grasp this truth. **This power we received is the Holy Spirit. The same Spirit that raised Jesus Christ from the dead lives in you... This strength is The absolute power!**

God wants you to prosper in all respects, including your psychological, emotional, and physical freedom. Since God wants your life to glorify Him, He asks you to use the weapons He placed at your disposal to win the wars that Satan tries to wage against you. It is time to use them, don't you think?

To further explain what you received as a gift, here's the definition of the word "power". It is literally translated as "authority" in Greek. It is written in *Colossians 1:13* that

you have been delive-
red for the power of
darkness; that means
that when you became
a child of God, you
have nothing to fear
from the authority of
darkness. The power
of darkness has no

> *You must realize that you received supernatural power when you became a child of God.*

hold on you and you are in a position of authority over the enemy, because you are now in Jesus Christ.

> *"The eyes of your understanding being enlightened; that ye may know what is the hope of his calling, and what the riches of the glory of his inheritance in the saints. And what is the exceeding greatness of his power to us-ward who believe, according to the working of his mighty power.* **Which he wrought in Christ, when he raised him from the dead, and set him at his own right hand in the heavenly places. Far above all principality, and power, and might, and dominion, and every name that is named, not only in this world, but also in that which is to come. And hath put all things under his feet,** *and gave him to be the head over all things to the church. Which is his body, the fulness of him that filleth all in all."*
>
> *Ephesians 1:18-23*

"Even when we were dead in sins, hath quickened us together with Christ, (by grace ye are saved). **And hath raised us up together, and made us sit together in heavenly places in Christ Jesus.** *That in the ages to come he might shew the exceeding riches of his grace in his kindness toward us through Christ Jesus."*

Ephesians 2:5-7

Everything becomes clearer! We are now seated with Jesus Christ in heavenly places and sitting above all principality, power, might, dominion and every name that is named. Hallelujah!

In the Greek, the Authority You Received Is Defined By Five Powers

FIRST POWER: DUNAMIS

The word "Dunamis" is translated as "dynamite". Some verses mention that we received a "power", which means, "dynamite". (*Acts 1:8*) It restores your life and "blasts" all the plans the enemy had plot against. It's the virtue (power) of God flowing through you to perform miracles and overthrow the enemy. Hallelujah!

SECOND POWER: EXOUSIA

The Exousia means "Delegated authority". We see this type of power in these two verses:

> *"And they were all amazed, insomuch that they questioned among themselves, saying, What thing is this? what new doctrine is this? for with authority commandeth he even the unclean spirits, and they do obey him."* Mark 1:27

> *"Then he called his twelve disciples together, and gave them power and authority over all devils, and to cure diseases."*
>
> *Luke 9:1*

This delegated authority gives us the strength to cast out demons, heal the sick, and perform signs and wonders in the name of Jesus Christ. The power you have within yourself, the "Exousia," gives you the supreme authority to command every torment to leave you, and it must leave! This authority gives you the power to order the fat on your body to melt, and it must melt. It gives you the power to command the imperfections on your body (varicose veins, cellulite...) to leave, and it's done, since the enemy created them.

THIRD POWER: ENERGIA

This power means "the energy of God" that's within you. Satan is a liar! No "burnout" can develop when you understand that you received the "Energia"! This power is also manifested through praise and worship. We feel the "energy" of God's presence. The "Energia" is also the force of propulsion manifested when we need more audacity to walk by faith, or face certain situations that intimidate us. When the situation is overcoming you or beyond your strength, it is the strength of God that takes charge, the "Energia" to lift you up. It is when we are weak that we are strong. Hallelujah!

FOURTH POWER: ISHUS

The "Ishus" is the force, the work, according to the authority received, the power of God received to resist temptation and deal with situations that seem bigger than us. If, by your own strength, you can't resist the temptations of gluttony, self-hatred, attacks of the enemy aimed at discouraging you, as well as lies and doubts of Satan, the "Ishus" in you will give you the strength to say no when you must say no! It's the "Ishus" that brings the necessary strength and endurance to get through this 777 Program and implement the revelations brought forth in this book.

FIFTH POWER: KRATOS

The fifth power you received is domination. The "Kratos" is the authority which puts you above all dominations from the powers of darkness, above the words "overweight", "torment", "obesity", "anorexia", "bulimia", "low self-esteem"... You are above all the enemy wanted to inflict upon your life to destroy you. You received the power to dominate over the forces of darkness. The power of God acts in you to destroy the works of the devil in your life and in the lives of others.

"I can do all things through Christ which strengtheneth me."

Philippians 4:13

160

You Received All Five Powers!

Now, use the five powers that you received. The authority has been delegated to you, in the name of Jesus Christ. Do you think that this authority was only intended for the apostles, prophets, evangelists, pastors, teachers, and doctors of the law? No! This authority is given through the baptism of the Holy Spirit and can be released through all who believe.

> *"And these signs shall follow **them that believe**; In my name shall they cast out devils; they shall speak with new tongues. They shall take up serpents; and if they drink any deadly thing, it shall not hurt them; they shall lay hands on the sick, and they shall recover."*
>
> *Mark 16:17*

Just Believe

Jesus is clear. He said: "And these signs shall follow them that believe ..." *(Mark 16:15-20)*, all you need is to believe. It will be done according to your faith... If you are a child of God, born again, you have the authority in the name of Jesus Christ to cast out demons; lay hands on the sick and they will be healed.

You also have the authority to lay hands on yourself and be delivered from the torments related to food and be healed of obesity, being overweight and any self-hatred. You received the power to say no to the enemy, to expel him from your mind (thoughts, emotions, will) and your body. You have control over your life, your spirit, your soul and your body.

It's truly the Lord's will that you use this weapon that was delegated to you, which is to take authority and release the five powers that are within you to achieve absolute victory!

Do Not Do As I Did For Many Years...

Here is what I did for approximately ten years: "Ah! Lord! Please, save me from the power food has over me. Deliver me from my obsessive thoughts about food. Make me lose weight... I don't want to be fat... I don't want to have hang-ups..."

One day, while reading the Bible, I realized two things: The first was that I didn't receive because I didn't ask correctly (*James 4:3*). And the second was that I was not using the authority I received. **It is written that whatever we would ask in the name of Jesus Christ, He would do it** (*John 14.13-14*). It's written that in His name, we would do greater things than Him.

Use Your Authority

Few Christians understand and use the name of Jesus Christ to change their situation. They cry for years and do not use the authority they received in the name of Jesus Christ.

> *From now on, you must release the authority on yourself and for yourself.*

From now on, you must release this authority on yourself and for yourself. You are entitled to it... Yes, you are indeed! These weapons you received are not just for others; they're for you as well, and they will give you victory. Your life must glorify God in every respect. Arise! The "Ishus", the "Dunamis", the "Exousia," the "Energia" and the "Kratos" are just waiting to be released for your benefit, your absolute victory, and your happiness.

Go! You're more than only a man or a woman! You're born again in Jesus Christ. You are a new born again creature, an ambassador of the Kingdom of God, and more than a conqueror. You are ready to conquer and overcome!

Say This Prayer:

Lord Jesus,

I come before you on this day. I thank you for everything you have done: you paid the price at the cross to make me free.

I received your complete salvation, which means that I am healed, delivered, made whole and supernaturally protected. I praise you and thank you Lord Jesus.

On this day, all of Satan's plans are broken in the name of Jesus Christ. Thank you Lord for showing me in advance the plans of the enemy and giving me your wisdom Holy Spirit to rebuke and break them.

I have decided to reject any spirit of gluttony, overeating, and any spirit of torment about food. I've decided to reject it today, once again in the name of Jesus Christ.

I have victory! I have dominion over unclean spirits. I have the authority over the enemy, and in the name of Jesus Christ, I command you, unclean spirit of temptation, to leave my life.

Hallelujah! Lord, I thank you because my body is getting firmer. I command my body to get firmer. I command my body to become more and more beautiful. I command my body to return to its initial weight, as you intended it to be, Lord.

Body, you restore yourself in the name of Jesus Christ. Varicose veins, you disappear in the name of Jesus Christ. Skin, you get firmer and replenished in the name of Jesus Christ.

Every disease and every weapon formed against me by the spirit of gluttony, such as hypoglycemia, diabetes, heart problem, or any other disease, I command you, in the powerful name of Jesus Christ, to come out of my life and never return.

This day is blessed. I decree it. Today, I succeed in everything I do. I am blessed going in and blessed going out.

I feel good with everyone I meet. I feel good with my body, my will, my emotions and my thoughts.

In the name of Jesus Christ. Amen!

Applying the Principles

- Refuse the temptation of overeating (gluttony).

- Be aware of the authority that was given to you and use it consistently at every moment! The Spirit that raised Jesus Christ from the dead lives in you.

- Learn to release the five powers and command to your soul and your body to be free and slim.

- Believe in God! Have faith!

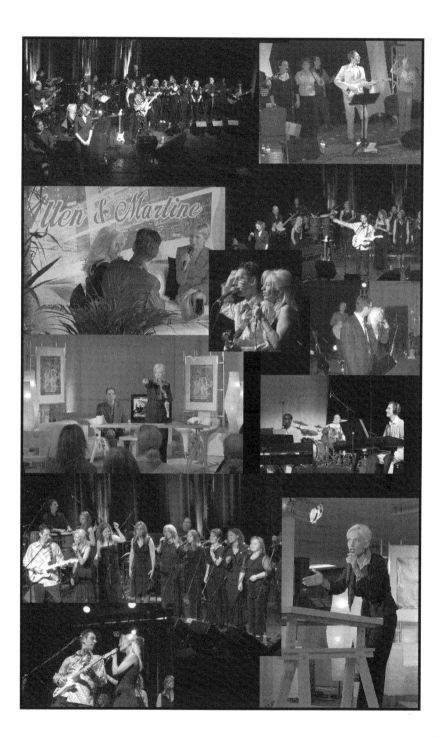

The Power of Your Words

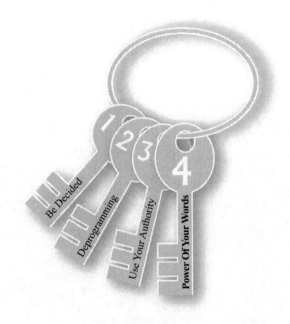

"Your future is in your mouth."

THE POWER OF YOUR TONGUE

"Death and life are in the power of the tongue: *and they that love it shall eat the fruit thereof."*

Proverbs 18:21

This key is the one Allen and I cherish in every details of our lives. It's a great revelation that you must grasp above everything! It had so much impact on our lives, and continues to do so!

We discovered a very powerful spiritual principle in the Word of God regarding words. They are powerful. The words we speak are of vital importance in our lives. They have consequences: good or bad.

> *The words we speak are of vital importance in our lives. They have consequences: good or bad.*

When God created humans, He gave us freedom to choose and express ourselves freely. We can choose our own words. **We are His only creation to have this capability.** No other creature (animals, angels...) has this opportunity. Angels can talk, but can only utter the words that God puts in their mouths. They act, but only after receiving orders from God..

169

God Said...

We find that the following sentence is written ten times in the first chapter of Genesis: **"God said..."** **Every time God spoke, the Holy Spirit was moving and acting on the Word of God.** He creates, and according to the verse found in Hebrews 1:3: *"...(He is) upholding all things by the word of his power,...."* Once God opens His mouth, His word becomes truth.

> *"So shall my word be that goeth forth out of my mouth: it shall not return unto me void, but it shall accomplish that which I please, and it shall prosper in the thing whereto I sent it."*
>
> *Isaiah 55:11*

Human Beings Were Created In God's Image

Adam and Eve were created in the image of God, of the same kind and therefore, had their own will. They had full authority to rule over and dominate every living creature on earth (over animals, nature, but not over man and woman). They had to rule by using their words. Their words would carry the power and anointing of God that was in them the moment they were created.

*"And God said, **Let us make man in our image**, after our likeness: and let them have dominion over the fish of the sea, and over the fowl of the air, and over the cattle, and over all the earth, and over every creeping thing that creepeth upon the earth. So God created man **in his own image, in the image of God created he him; male and female created he them.***

***And God blessed them, and God said unto them, Be fruitful, and multiply, and replenish the earth, and subdue it: and have dominion over the fish of the sea, and over the fowl of the air, and over every living thing that moveth upon the earth.** And God said, Behold, I have given you every herb bearing seed, which is upon the face of all the earth, and every tree, in the which is the fruit of a tree yielding seed; to you it shall be for meat.*

And to every beast of the earth, and to every fowl of the air, and to every thing that creepeth upon the earth, wherein there is life, I have given every green herb for meat: and it was so."

Genesis 1:26-30

The Offensive Weapon: Your Words

The foundation of all our weapons as a believer is the sword of the Spirit, which is the Word of God (*Ephesiens 6:17*). Jesus was the living Word of God manifested in the flesh.

> *"And the Word was made flesh, and dwelt among us, (and we beheld his glory, the glory as of the only begotten of the Father,) full of grace and truth."*
>
> John 1:14

Then, God gave the written Word, the Gospel, in order for us to use it to be victorious in our everyday lives. This sword, the Word of God, is ours to use to defend our rights as born again children of God, and to live a victorious life, in the abundance that Jesus came to give us. Jesus Christ himself used the Word of God to rebuke Satan's temptation in the desert.

> *"And Jesus being full of the Holy Ghost returned from Jordan, and was led by the Spirit into the wilderness. Being forty days tempted of the devil. And in those days he did eat nothing: and when they were ended, he afterward hungered. And the devil said unto him, If thou be the Son of God, command this stone that it be made bread.*
>
> ***And Jesus answered him, saying, It is written:*** *That man shall not live by bread alone, but by every word of God. And the devil, taking him up into an high mountain, shewed unto him all the kingdoms of the world in a moment of time. And the devil said unto him, All this power will I give thee, and the glory of them: for that is delivered unto me; and to whomsoever I will*

I give it. If thou therefore wilt worship me, all shall be thine.

And Jesus answered and said unto him, *Get thee behind me, Satan: for it is written: Thou shalt worship the Lord thy God, and him only shalt thou serve. And he brought him to Jerusalem, and set him on a pinnacle of the temple, and said unto him, If thou be the Son of God, cast thyself down from hence: For it is written, He shall give his angels charge over thee, to keep thee: And in their hands they shall bear thee up, lest at any time thou dash thy foot against a stone.*

And Jesus answering said unto him: *It is said, Thou shalt not tempt the Lord thy God.*

And when the devil had ended all the temptation, he departed from him for a season."

Luke 4:1-13

> **Learn to release the Word of God through your mouth.**

To live this life of joy and take back what Satan came to steal from your life, you must use this powerful weapon. Learn to release the Word of God through your mouth. It is an essential key to your victory. At the end of this book, you will find a few verses on the power of the Word. Read them and meditate on them. You will continue to be deprogrammed of viruses and move on toward your absolute victory!

You Can Either Bless or Curse Yourself Through Your Mouth

*"**Out of the same mouth proceedeth blessing and cursing.** My brethren, these things ought not so to be. Doth a fountain send forth at the same place sweet water and bitter? Can the fig tree, my brethren, bear olive berries? either a vine, figs? so can no fountain both yield salt water and fresh."*

James 3:10-12

You can either be blessed or cursed through your mouth. How often have you released curse-containing words upon your life? How often have you declared you would be gaining weight, even before eating?

- Hey! Anything makes me gain weight...
- I'll get fat if I eat this...
- I just look at chocolate and I gain weight...
- I can't help it, it's in my genes...
- I'll never succeed...

Your life is the result of words you have spoken about yourself. How many words of this kind have you spoken about yourself, against you and your body? Now, start proclamation the blessing on yourself. Start saying: "Thank you Lord, I eat without depriving myself, until I am not hungry anymore and my body comes back to its perfect shape. Thank you Lord, my body is restored as you have created it when you formed me in my mother's womb."

174

Your Language Is The Deciding Factor For Your Body and Your Emotions

You have God's authority to release words of truth from your mouth, which are words of victory.

Your mouth has the power to change your situation regarding food and your body, because you were created in God's image and He created everything by His Word. You are the captain of your ship; you turn the rudder of the boat by your words. You have **God's authority** to release words of truth from your mouth, which are words of victory.

For example: we can see the impact words have when conjugal violence occurs. In most cases, we know that the first form of violence is verbal and/or psychological abuse. The words spoken can negatively affect self-esteem and have a destructive impact on people's lives, and the perception they have of themselves. We must reject these words and confront them by repeating the Word of God.

Here's another example: Mr. Donald Trump, a very prosper real estate businessman. I've learned that Donald Trump's father kept repeating that everything his son was touching turned to gold. That is exactly what his life now reflects. Although at times he's gone through dire financial times, until now, he managed to get out of these situations. His soul is "very muscular" in this area because of words of financial prosperity repeated over and over again about his financial success.

We've just seen two very different examples: One in which words can destroy and annihilate the person, and the other in which the words conveyed were positive words of prosperity. Of course, we are not all born in the same soil. For some, it will be necessary to persevere in order to obtain what they want to see happen, but the Word of God does not come back void.

Satan Is The Liar Who Plays With Your Thoughts

Satan knows the power words have on human beings and he needs our mouth to destroy us, while God wants to use it to bless us. The enemy's strategy is to sow evil or negative thoughts in our minds. He knows very well that they will defile our soul and end up coming out as destructive words. The devil uses what he's sown in our minds (our thoughts, emotions) to make us sin by our words. This is how Satan works in people's lives. The thought is repeated in your mind until it's fully embedded. These words eventually come out of your mind, and wind up in your mouth, bypassing your thought process.

*"... **for out of the abundance of the heart the mouth speaketh.** A good man out of the good treasure of the heart bringeth forth good things: and an evil man out of the evil treasure bringeth forth evil things."*

Matthew 12:34-35

Since birth, you've been accustomed to speaking negatively in several areas of your life. **Unconsciously, in every day conversations, you use the terms failure and death to talk about the beauty of your body, your personality, your emotions and your perceptions about food...** People ask themselves why they fail to lose weight and stay slim, but when I hear them talk, I understand everything. By the words of their mouth, they prevent God from acting in their lives.

> People ask themselves why they fail to lose weight and stay slim, but when I hear them talk, I understand everything. **By the words of their mouth, they prevent God from acting in their lives.**

The Word of God In Your Heart

You need God's Word in abundance in your heart, God's will in your mouth and you'll see your destiny change. The destiny that God has in store for you will be accomplished. As your words gave permission to Satan to intervene in your life, your body, and your relationship with food, your words can now unleash God's powerful intervention. The Word of God you release will bring healing, restoration, deliverance, and freedom.

By knowing that your tongue has an impact on your body and on the way you feed yourself, you will be able to put a stop to **Satan's works. You will then be able to dominate and censor Satan by learning to control your own tongue. Your tongue is only an instrument. The key is in your heart...** What is in abundance in your heart will come out of your mouth. If your heart is filled with the Word of God and His will for you, it will come out of your mouth. You will then use the authority of the Word of God to break the power of the words you expressed in the past. Fill your heart with the Word of God and that's exactly what will be released. The works of God will be accomplished by force of circumstance. You will express what is in abundance in your heart. Start today to build the body you want and the freedom to which you aspire.

Satan Will No Longer Use Your Mouth Against Your Body

Satan was using your tongue to inflame the course of your life. You were possibly programmed from birth to talk negatively about your life, your body, and how you feed yourself...

Now stop and observe how you talk about yourself, your body, and food. Make a habit of listening to your own words. Notice the impact they have on your life. You will make very interesting and constructive discoveries through this new journey. You are being transformed! Work on the way you talk about yourself.

Even if you do not believe it at first, by proclaiming God's truth, you will finally believe it as you begin to perceive the changes, as minimal as they are. Negative thoughts will be replaced by words of truth and life. The power of God will then be manifested in your life. Your destiny will be filled with joy and freedom.

You must know that you should not condemn yourself if you say a negative word contrary to the will and Word of God! Simply repent to the Lord for what you just said. Break that word in the name of Jesus Christ and replace it with God's truth.

Remember that if you proclaim the truth through your mouth, the truth will set you free. Do not expect any change to happen about your problems without the Word of God in your mouth.

Work on the way you talk about yourself.

Say This Prayer:

Heavenly Father,

In the name of Jesus, I make the right decision to control my mouth. I renounce, reject and repent of every word uttered against You and Your work in my life.

I cancel the power of those negative words and I sanctify my mouth to express Your Word, which is the Truth.

I get into the habit of speaking in accordance with the Word of God. As Your child, I confess that I am healed, slim, delivered, and filled by your powerful Holy Spirit.

I have victory over my emotions and my body because you wanted it to be so. Father, I thank you that the words of my mouth do not contradict my thoughts anymore, in the name of Jesus Christ.

Father, in the name of Jesus Christ, I make the right decision to control my mouth. Thank you Lord for the marvelous creation that I am.

I cancel now in the name of Jesus Christ all the words that I said against my body and my dietary freedom. All the words of fear, of hatred, of rejection and destruction are canceled in the name of Jesus Christ.

I release that my body is getting more beautiful and that I am free in my relationship with food. I eat what I want when I am hungry and my body comes back in shape, as you created it. I feel good with my body and my relationship with food; I am slim and beautiful.

In the name of Jesus Christ. Amen!

Applying the Principles

In the next 49 days of the 777 Program, I would urge you to repeat this sentence out loud, at least three times a day before eating:

"Thank you Lord for the marvelous creation that I am. My body will restore itself like you originally created it. I eat and I stop when I'm full. I'm slim and beautiful and I'm at peace with food."

- Make a list of all the negative words that were said about you and **that you accepted and in turn, repeated** to sabotage your self-esteem and destroy your body image.

- Take authority over these words! Break them in the name of Jesus Christ and declare the truth according to the Word of God.

- Stop and look at how you talk about yourself, your body, and food. Make it a habit of listening to your own words. Note the impact they have on your life. Enhance your self-esteem through biblical truths. Even if you don't believe it, by repeating the truth of the Word of God on yourself, you'll eventually believe it. The words of life and the power of God will then be manifested in your life. Your destiny will be filled with joy and freedom!

If the devil tries to tempt you with all sorts of negative thoughts in front of the mirror, stop him from robbing you! Do the following:

- Stop looking at yourself in the mirror for a few seconds, then...

- Say out loud: "I praise you Lord, I'm fearfully and wonderfully made, a marvelous creation indeed. I am slim and I feel good about my body."

- Repeat it several times until you feel your soul lighten up by the truth of God.

- Next, if you wish, return to the mirror and you'll see that your perception of yourself has changed. You will see the improvements the Holy Spirit is undertaking in your soul and your body, rather than look at what the enemy wants you to see.

Fifth Week

5ᵀᴴ Key:

Applying
the 3 Spiritual Weapons

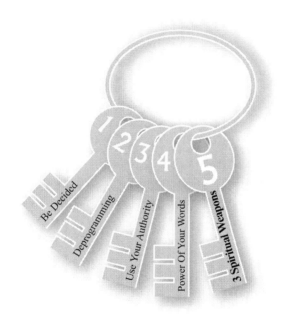

*"The rifle is useless to the soldier
if he doesn't use it."*

APPLYING THE SPIRITUAL WEAPONS

*Y*ou are soldiers of God bearing spiritual weapons. Throughout this book, you are being strengthened as a child of God. You are able to see a progression in your life's journey. As you realize who you are in Jesus Christ, and what the real fight is about, you are becoming stronger. With this fifth key, you will be able to understand and **use powerful spiritual weapons: prayer, fasting and sowing. I will only do an overview of these three weapons, because I could write a book about each of them. If I mention them, it is because they are important and often neglected, or misused by the children of God.**

God has provided us with powerful tools to effectively fight against Satan and his kingdom, but we must use them. Depending on the fight you have to undertake, God has given you different weapons. It is important to understand that the war you have to win is not carnal, but spiritual. Here is what the Word of God confirms:

> **"For we wrestle not against flesh and blood,** *but against principalities, against powers, against the rulers of the darkness of this world, against spiritual wickedness in high places."*
>
> *Ephesians 6:12*

186

"For though we walk in the flesh, we do not war after the flesh. For the weapons of our warfare are not carnal, but mighty through God to the pulling down of strong holds."

2 Corinthians 10:3-4

Three Targeted Weapons For This Fight:

1. Prayer

2. Fasting

3. Sowing

This key will enable you to face your spiritual enemy and defeat him! The fourth key taught you how to use the Word of God, which is the sword of the Holy Spirit. In Ephesians 6:13-18, we find the weapons that God gives us. Reading these verses is not sufficient; you must apply them in your everyday lives. The weapons I am talking about; prayer, fasting, and sowing, are other weapons you can consistently use to come out victorious over torments about food and/or obesity. For the child of God, these are powerful tools to use to overturn strongholds by the virtue of God.

How many people have had their lives transformed simply because they put into action the Word of God?

How many people have had their lives transformed simply because they put into action the Word of God? It is not sufficient to simply hear it and go on as if we learned anything.

> *"**But be ye doers of the word,** and not hearers only, deceiving your own selves. For if any be a hearer of the word, and not a doer, he is like unto a man beholding his natural face in a glass. For he beholdeth himself, and goeth his way, and straightway forgetteth what manner of man he was. **But whoso looketh into the perfect law of liberty, and continueth therein, he being not a forgetful hearer, but a doer of the work, this man shall be blessed in his deed."***

> *James 1:22-25*

If you want to have an impact on your freedom and your weight, this teaching will enable you to obtain the desired victory. The closer we get to God, the more we are shielded against the enemy. When we praise God, His glory comes down on us and He responds to our requests. For this to happen, we must apply and put into practice the Word of God. The enemy has no choice but to flee if you use all the weapons, especially prayer, fasting and sowing. The strongholds Satan has on you will crumble in the name of Jesus Christ! Overturn the arguments that are not of God, those that Satan tries to put in your mind to prevent you form walking in your freedom and to keep you captive with your excess weight.

188

*"Casting down imaginations, and every high thing that exalteth itself against the knowledge of God, **and bringing into captivity every thought to the obedience of Christ."***

2 Corinthians 10:5

The more you obey the Word of God and put it into practice in every detail of your life, the more you become an invincible fortress to the enemy.

Do not let him play with your thoughts and perceptions anymore. Assert yourself as a child of God: "I am beautiful ... I am slim, etc." You are free in the name of Jesus Christ! If some days seem harder than others, bring your thoughts captive onto God.

The more you obey the Word of God and put it into practice in every aspect of your life, the more you become an invincible fortress to the enemy.

First Targeted Weapon For Battle:

Prayer

Many of you know about prayer. Here are some verses to read and reread to understand what God wants to bring us:

> *"And it shall come to pass, that before they call, I will answer; and while they are yet speaking, I will hear."*
>
> Isaiah 65:24

> *"He shall call upon me, and I will answer him: I will be with him in trouble; I will deliver him, and honour him."*
>
> Psalms 91:15

> *"Call unto me, and I will answer thee, and show thee great and mighty things, which thou knowest not."*
>
> Jeremiah 33:3

> *"Ask, and it shall be given you; seek, and ye shall find; knock, and it shall be opened unto you: For every one that asketh receiveth; and he that seeketh findeth; and to him that knocketh it shall be opened."*
>
> Matthew 7:7-8

190

"And all things, whatsoever ye shall ask in prayer, believing, ye shall receive."

Matthew 21:22

"And whatsoever ye shall ask in my name, that will I do, that the Father may be glorified in the Son."

John 14:13

"If ye abide in me, and my words abide in you, ye shall ask what ye will, and it shall be done unto you."

John 15:7

"And whatsoever we ask, we receive of him, because we keep his commandments, and do those things that are pleasing in his sight."

1 John 3:22

The Power of Prayer

If you ask God in faith, He will grant it to you. It is already accomplished. Believe that you received it... Ask and you shall receive: seek and you shall find... How many times have you asked the Lord to take away your cellulite, your excess weight?

How many times have you prayed for your body to change? How many times have you said to God: "Lord, I thank you. I am a marvelous creation! Your works are wonderful and you make me even more beautiful."

Jesus said that you do not receive because you do not ask or you do not know how to ask. You must pray in the name of Jesus Christ by

Prayer is powerful to overthrow strongholds!

decreeing what you want to see happen for you. You must pray with authority, with truth according to the Word of God, and you must do this constantly in your heart. Make it a routine to pray. Stop a moment to welcome the Holy Spirit. Thank the Lord for all He has done and what He is currently doing in your life. God often works in the background. Perhaps you don't see His glory yet, but your miracle is on its way! Declare in the name of Jesus Christ what you want to see accomplished for yourself and you will see it! Prayer is powerful to put down strongholds. When you know how to ask, decree it and release the Word of God in your life; you will receive over and above whatever you ask. To regain your slenderness, pray as often as possible. Pray before eating... Say this: "Thank you Lord for this food. Holy Spirit, show me when I am no longer hungry and give me the strength to stop eating at that point, in the name of Jesus Christ. Amen!" You will starve the spirit of gluttony to death! Be free!

In the story of the widow, Jesus shows us the importance of being persistent in prayer until we get what we ask *(Luke 18:3)*. This story shows us how this woman went before the judge for justice. He did not care much about her. However, through perseverance, she succeeded. It's up to you to obtain justice either with your freedom or your weight!

You do not have to pay the price of previous generations. Jesus Christ paid it at the cross for you! Then return to God and say: "Thank you Lord! What I ask of you, I believe I've received it. I ask you and it's accomplished!"

Persevere! Do as the widow to get what you desire! Pray! The Lord will answer. It's truly a powerful weapon to put into practice. Constantly talk to the Lord and the results won't wait. If you are about to eat or open the fridge... Pray constantly and ask the Holy Spirit's help. It is a vital key within the fifth key.

Receiving means taking by force.

Let the Holy Spirit Intercede For You

The Holy Spirit can help you conquer the enemy. Moreover, it is written:

> *"Then he answered and spake unto me, saying, This is the word of the Lord unto Zerubbabel, saying, **Not by might, nor by power, but by my spirit, saith the Lord of hosts.**"*
>
>

Zechariah 4:6

> *"**Likewise the Spirit also helpeth our infirmities:** for we know not what we should pray for as we ought: but the Spirit itself maketh intercession for us with groanings which cannot be uttered."*
>
>

Romans 8:26

If it happens that you do not know how to pray anymore or if you feel weak, discouraged, about to abandon, the Holy Spirit will help you. Let Him intercede for you and through you. Say: "Holy Spirit, thank you for interceding for me to find back my perfect weight, to have better self-esteem, stop sinning by overeating, etc." Those who received the baptism of the Holy Spirit must pray in tongues out loud every day to let Him intercede through your mouth. He will strengthen your soul. In asking for His help, do not be surprised to see the torments eliminated and obtain revelations. The Holy Spirit will show you the path to take to achieve your victory. He will give you revelations. He will guide you, edify you, teach you, lift you up, exhort you and correct you.

God said that He has clothed us with His power, but we must use that power for something to happen. The Holy Spirit was sent by Jesus Christ for you. He is in your life on earth to glorify God, so He can and will work miracles through your body. He knows what to say to your soul to strengthen and fortify it. He knows how to intercede to the Heavenly Father to bring down the fortresses of the enemy. We do not only have a God of weekends, but a God of everyday, living in our body. He gave us the Holy Spirit to make us strong when we're weak *(Zechariah 4:6)*. When the enemy wants to knock you down, the Holy Spirit begins to intercede for you. If your emotions pull you down, it's through the Spirit of God that you'll pick yourself up. He was sent to be our Helper. He is our support for victory in every area of our lives. He guides us, teaches us, strengthens us, and shows us hidden things.

Pray constantly in your heart and regularly in tongues, out loud! Do not wait until you are in a state of distress to ask for the Lord's help. Always be consistent and perseverant. The Lord calls His people to live a victorious life. Do not take a step forward and two steps backwards!

With God, we go forward, and forward, and forward!

195

Second Targeted Weapon For Combat:

Fasting

I fasted a lot and I still do. **I'm often surprised to see that God's children don't fast. The power of fasting is so strong!** This must become a lifestyle for Christians. We get a lot of physical and spiritual healing through fasting. Several Christians who practice fasting testify about its benefits. God works mightily when we submit ourselves to it. His presence becomes stronger. It is a powerful weapon! We stop feeding our flesh to feed our spirit by the presence and power of God. We must not do it to lose weight even if we will inevitably become slimmer by doing so. **There is a big difference between spiritual fasting and the world's fasting.**

Prayer and reading the Word of God, combined with fasting, becomes our spiritual food. They give us extraordinary strength to stand firm against the enemy. They are mandatory to build up our soul during

> *We stop feeding our flesh to feed our spirit by the presence and power of God.*

this period of making our flesh die. Fasting is a powerful weapon, specifically against eating disorders and excess weight. Surely, with this weapon, you are "starving to death" what came against your freedom and your slenderness.

Why Fast? Here Are the Reasons:

- It's a very powerful spiritual weapon.
- It appears in the Old and New Testaments and God's people practice it.
- It brings you closer to God.
- It slays your flesh, cleanses your soul, and helps you to hear what the Holy Spirit has to say.

By fasting, we operate by the Spirit and not the flesh. The flesh is death; the Spirit is life.

"Therefore, brethren, we are debtors, not to the flesh, to live after the flesh. For if ye live after the flesh, ye shall die: but if ye through the Spirit do mortify the deeds of the body, ye shall live. For as many as are led by the Spirit of God, they are the sons of God. For ye have not received the spirit of bondage again to fear; but ye have received the Spirit of adoption, whereby we cry, Abba, Father!"

Romans 8:12-15

You separate yourself from your flesh... So, generally you also abstain from sexual activity... You take a step closer to God. This makes a lot of difference, since fasting cleanses your soul and brings revelations. Fasting brings more than weight loss or the melting of cellulite. What are the benefits?

- Increased power from the Holy Spirit
- Breaking of spiritual ties (patterns)
- Capacity to cope with something that seems bigger for you
- Increased presence of God
- Calling/consecration for ministry (time set apart for this purpose)
- Clearer discernment of God's will
- Breaking of the spirit of dependence
- Physical and emotional healing
- Body detoxification

If wrestling with food seems more difficult on certain days, use this powerful weapon to defeat the enemy. You'll destroy him! When I felt that the enemy sought to undermine me, I took authority over him: "You want me to eat by gluttony? I'm fasting then!" Immediately, I felt I had the upper hand over Satan. Bring down the fortresses of the enemy with this powerful weapon! Obtaining physical healings can fortify your soul. The more you include fasting to your lifestyle, the more you will get the results mentioned above. You can't help but see your body change. Be determined to achieve victory! Fasting is biblical: Jesus fasted for forty days, as for Moses, he fasted twice for forty days; Elijah... Daniel... Closer in time, Abraham Lincoln had declared a national fast when he was President of the United States to achieve victories for his country. Participants included those who believed and wanted to see the hand of God move mightily.

Receive your deliverance also! You are on the battlefield... Fight with your spiritual weapons, including this one. Take action and receive complete restoration for your body. It is a powerful tool to conquer something. You will be amazed at how much you regain your strength and energy. I have often heard Christians say they didn't until they heard the Lord tell them to do so. Well, I can tell you that these people who did not fast often in their life have not experienced many victories. The apostle Paul said it well: "Seize the weapons to stand against the wiles of the devil." Spiritual weapons are available to us. Do you foresee an attack? Seize the appropriate weapon to defeat Satan's plans.

> *Don't wait until you feel like fasting or feel ready to fast. I can assure you that what's coming against you has absolutely no desire for you to fast.*

The devil will be playing with your mind to prevent you from seizing the weapon that will destroy him. He instills all sorts of reasons in your mind...

Here Are Some Examples of Thoughts Planted By the Enemy:

- I can't fast; I will be too weak to work.
- What will people say if they see me fast?
- I do not have enough will, I will fail.
- I become aggressive when I fast, so I do not fast anymore.
- I am cooking food for my family... It is too difficult to not eat.
- It is not necessary to fast... I only have to pray.

Yet, as a child of God, I can tell you that fasting is an integral part of our lifestyle. It is of the utmost importance if we wish to obtain true victories. Fasting is a powerful weapon to defeat the plans of Satan against your body (weight loss, health) and towards your soul (torments, relationship with God, etc..). Jesus Christ Himself told the disciples of John the Baptist that they would fast when He would be gone.

> *"And they said unto him, Why do the disciples of John fast often, and make prayers, and likewise the disciples of the Pharisees; but thine eat and drink?*
>
> *And he said unto them, Can ye make the children of the bridechamber fast, while the bridegroom is with them?* ***But the days will come, when the bridegroom shall be taken away from them, and then shall they fast in those days."***
>
> Luke 5:33-35

What Type of Fast Would You Like to Do? There Are Three Types:

- Absolute, without water, like Moses' fast
- Normal: with water or juice
- Partial: skip a meal.../fruits and vegetables.../go without treats...

I would advise you to start slowly, especially if you have never fasted. You can start with a partial fast by skipping a meal, eating only fruits or vegetables or, by depriving yourself of a few treats during the day, then two, then three...

Generally, most people do a normal fast. This means that you only drink liquids (water, fruit juice or vegetable juice) and don't eat solid food. The total fast, i.e. without liquid and water is rarely used. If you don't know what kind of fast you should do, ask the Lord. It is sometimes better to make a little commitment and follow through before God rather than seeing too big and not be able to follow through with your promise. What is important is to start and slowly increase the number of days you fast. You will see transformations happen in your life.

After having fasted a few times for 24 hours, I suggest you do regular three-day fasts (three days and three nights) throughout the 777 Program. The three-day fast is particularly good for breaking generational ties and the spirit of dependence.

Recommendations:

3 Days Of Fasting Per Week For 7 Weeks
Or
21 Days Of Consecutive Fasting.

Is there a situation that's not budging in your life? Do you want revelations in your life? Then fast!

Third Targeted Weapon For Combat:

Sowing

This story deeply touched me: I heard the story of a pastor who preaches around the world. Returning from an evangelism trip in Russia, he found his wife in tears. He asked her why she was crying and she replied: "*Look at your son and call him.*" He was three years old, and was playing without taking notice of his surroundings. The father called his son, clapped his hands... No reaction! He stood before him: the child didn't seem to see him.

This well-known pastor preaches that God is powerful and that He still heals today. He was distraught. So, he decided to bring his son to the hospital to have him tested. A few hours later, a psychiatrist came to the pastor. "*Have you come for my son?*" He said. "*No, I'm here for you.*" "*Why?*" the pastor asked. The psychiatrist told him that his son had an IQ so high that it created an irreversible problem in his brain and he would never be able to learn anything. He would never speak. He would never live like a normal child. This is a very rare disease. He would be dependant on his father and mother for the rest of his days.

The pastor took his son and went back into his car. He began to cry out to God: "*Lord, I don't understand. I preach around the world. I see healings and miracles before my eyes and my son will never live normally? You promised me he would serve you. Satan wants to rob me of that promise.*

Lord, what should I do?" He did not let go of his promise. He refused to let the lies of the enemy have any hold on him. He refused the diagnosis that had been placed upon his son. He began to pray with his wife and cry to God: *"Lord, you promised me that my son would be serving you. Yes, he will speak one day and will call me daddy. I reject this lie! Tell me what to do!"* The Lord told him he should sow an amount for his son's recovery and by faith, believe that the seed would bring the desired harvest.

God asked something very big for this man, but he decided to obey Him. He did all in his power to collect the money in only a few weeks. God told him to sow that amount of money and he obeyed Him, as sowing is a principle, a powerful spiritual law. In the weeks that followed, his son began to recover supernaturally. This is a true story; the son is about 16 years old now and attends church with his father. At 12, he was already sharing his testimony. The enemy's diagnosis fell because the pastor connected himself with a powerful spiritual law and he had decided to obey the voice of God. He obtained his victory!

This story touched me deeply, and since then, I have been sowing for my body so I would be victorious as well. I've asked the Lord what should be the amount of my seed, and I obeyed Him. Everything is a matter of sowing and obedience... You can also win your battles using this powerful spiritual law.

> *Sowing is a principle, a powerful spiritual law.*

*"Be not deceived; God is not mocked: **for whatsoever a man soweth, that shall he also reap.**"*

Galatians 6:7

God created everything with a seed:

- The Word of God is a seed;
- Our words are a seed;
- Vegetation is propagated by a seed;
- Humans reproduce with a seed.

Sow what you want to receive; Here are a few examples:

- Your relationship with the Lord: Draw near to Him and He will draw near to you;
- Your friendships: Be a true friend in order to have good friends;
- Your love: Sow love and you will harvest love;
- Your financial investments: Sow in your investments and you will reap more money;
- Your health: Nutrition, exercises ...

If I want friendship or love, I must sow to get friendship or love, etc. When we connect to God's laws and we ask: "Lord, what's the amount I should sow?" and we sow this amount, God responds to our requests. He is faithful to His Word. The impact on our lives is real.

204

Several verses refer to this:

> *"And he said, Unto you it is given to know the mysteries of the kingdom of God: but to others in parables; that seeing they might not see, and hearing they might not understand. Now the parable is this: The seed is the word of God. Those by the way side are they that hear; then cometh the devil, and taketh away the word out of their hearts, lest they should believe and be saved."*
>
> *Luke 8:10-12*

> *"Being born again, not of corruptible seed, but of incorruptible, by the word of God, which liveth and abideth for ever."*
>
> *1 Peter 1:23*

The Power of the Financial Seed into the Kingdom of God:

- Pours out on us a blessing in abundance (*Malachi 3:10-11*);
- Rebukes the devourer (*Malachi 3:11*)
- Give a name to your seed and you will see your harvest (*Galatians 6:7*);
- Give and you shall receive (*Luke 6:38*).

> **If I don't sow,
> I will reap nothing!**

If you want a harvest in your life, you need to sow and name your seed. In the Kingdom of God, everything is a matter of sowing and the types of soils in which to sow. If I do not sow, I will not reap! There are Christians who understand that they must give their tithe, but they sow it anywhere, in any ground, anyhow, in any amount. To connect with the spiritual laws of God, you must pay the tithe of 10% of your income as requested by the Lord, but also obey about the amounts that God may ask of you for specific victories. How much is He actually asking you for your victory?

As for me, when I asked Him the amount to sow to regain my slenderness, He asked me to fast and sow a certain amount. I planted this specific seed for my body in order to reap a specific harvest. I obeyed to His will…

And I received my harvest! To this day, I continue to apply this principle to other aspects of my life. I go from glory to glory!

If you truly want results in your life, and in this particular area, you absolutely need to connect to the spiritual laws of God. There are several ways to sow. Be specific in your requests! What crops do you want to harvest? If you plant carrot seeds, expect to see carrots grow.

When you sow into the Kingdom of God, ask what you want to see grow in your spiritual garden. If you put a seed

206

for physical deliverance about your weight, think about this pastor who planted for his son: he wanted his child to be healed. Do like him!

Do not sow in any soil without naming your harvest. Sow in a rich soil (a ministry bearing the fruits you want to see in your life) so it can grow! The favor of God will be deposited in that soil. Say: "Lord, I am sowing for this specific thing." Thereafter, take care of your spiritual garden. What happens when we don't take care of the soil? It becomes an untilled wasteland! The seeds die!

Water constantly your spiritual garden by your words and your prayers. You have to believe, as you believe that in planting carrot seeds, you will grow carrots.

Say This Prayer:

Lord,

I receive the best for myself. I pray for this wonderful day ahead. I welcome you Holy Spirit! Fill my life completely today.

I feel good in my own body. I have renounced the spirit of gluttony and I have absolute victory! Feed me spiritually during my fast. Nurture my soul with your presence.

My body is restored and supernaturally embellished. I receive the compliments that people give me with gratitude. I receive every good word and am going from glory to glory. I'm blessed today, and successful in everything I do, in the powerful name of Jesus Christ.

I sow in accordance with your will, Lord. I sow the amount you place in my heart with faith and obedience, in the soil you want and I harvest.

Lord, every door closed to me by the enemy, supernaturally opens by your mighty hand.

In the name of Jesus Christ. Amen!

(Pray in tongues for a few minutes and let the Holy Spirit intercede for you.)

Applying the Principles

- Continue to practice all the keys and the teachings you received since the beginning.

- Every day of the week, say a prayer addressing your specific needs.

- Fast with a goal that matches your needs and continue to use this weapon throughout the program. I suggest that you fast regularly during the coming weeks for 3 days per week during 7 weeks (a total of 21 days), or do a normal fast of 21 consecutive days.

- Pray in tongues a few minutes per day, every day. Pray in the shower, in the car, while shaving or putting on make-up...

- Ask the Lord for a specific amount to sow to get victory towards food and/ or your body, where to plant that seed, and claim your harvest everyday.

- Get a small notebook where you list all your seeds and keep your spiritual garden watered with prayers and the Word.

SIXTH WEEK

6TH KEY:

CRAVE FOR...

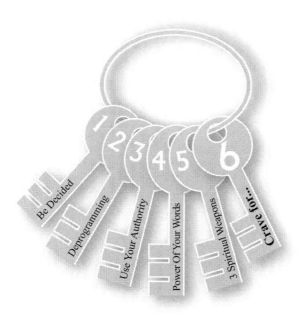

"When you remove something, you must to replace it with something else."

CRAVE FOR...

 here are three important things you must be hungry for aside from food. Food is essential, but only for one thing: your belly.

"Meats for the belly, and the belly for meats: but God shall destroy both it and them. Now the body is not for fornication, but for the Lord; and the Lord for the body."

1 Corinthians 6:13

However, your soul is craving three essential things that will cater to your sense of achievement, as well as your spiritual, psychological, emotional, and physical well-being: To be hungry for God, for yourself and for people who crave all you have to offer. The first and most important is:

1. Crave For God

"My soul thirsteth for God, for the living God."

Psalms 42:2a

We must learn to nourish our spirit, our soul, and therefore our bodies, with our relationship with the Lord. **This is the fundamental basis for complete deliverance.** We were created to have an intimate relationship with God. Without this relationship, we are deprived of seeing the glory of God manifested in our lives. The only thing that can nourish our souls and prevent us from eating our emotions is our relationship with Jesus Christ.

He is the Source; He is the daily bread our spirit and soul need. He fills all emptiness within us. The Lord must be the first person you call when things go wrong. Not the fridge, the cake, the bag of potato chips or someone else... **He's your Savior!** He can and will save you from any situation that is too difficult for you.

Food Does Not Fill Any Void

Based on my experience, I could not fill the void left by food. Certainly, my belly was full. I felt full, bloated and uncomfortable in my body, but still not satisfied. **The only one** able to set me free and **satisfy you as well is the Lord, and your relationship with Him.**

> *"And be not drunk with wine, wherein is excess; but be filled with the Spirit;"*
>
> *Ephesians 5:18*

It's so good to have intimacy with God! The Holy Spirit, who stands by your side, longs to have a real relationship with you and to fill you with His presence... And you? If you want to see your life step up to another level and see your body transformed, you must have this special relationship with the Holy Spirit. You must crave for God everyday. Your hunger and thirst for Him must become progressively more important. His increased presence in you will fill you when you feel rejected, lonely, sad, and angry... It is not food that will fill your pain anymore, but God's presence. You must have this passion, this craving for God.

Food will not fill your pain, but only God's presence will.

"Oh that men would praise the Lord for his goodness, and for his wonderful works to the children of men! For he satisfieth the longing soul, and filleth the hungry soul with goodness."

Psalms 107:8-9

Eat the Word of God

With God in your life, you can no longer remain lukewarm. You must be on fire for Him. His presence will fill any void. No void in your soul can be filled with food. Perhaps you felt unloved when you were young? You are probably lacking love and affection now? It is possible that nobody complimented you, uplifted you, or encouraged you... Perhaps you've been judged, or falsely accused? You probably haven't been recognized at your true worth, but only God can give you all this **perfectly**, and even more. He wants to fulfill you and bring you into the

No void in your soul can be filled with food.

214

perfect destiny He created you for. Turn to Him more than ever. Eat the Word of God and see His glory be manifested within you and your body

> *"But he answered and said, It is written, Man shall not live by bread alone, but by every word that proceedeth out of the mouth of God."*
>
> *Matthew 4:4*

As you live by the Word of God, you will see the supernatural in your life.

Anyone may disappoint you, but God will never disappoint you.

Remember that you can never be more prosperous than your soul. Inquiring and assimilating the Word of God, all the while developing your relationship with Him; these are the only ways your soul will prosper. **Your relationship with food must meet only the needs of your belly... That's all!** If you want to have this passionate relationship with Jesus Christ, be filled with the Holy Spirit, and not food, read on...

2. Crave For Yourself

"Thou shalt love thy neighbour as thyself."
Matthew 19:19b

> **You must immediately start to maximize your full potential.**

This chapter is an important revelation. It is essential that you learn to crave for what is within you, for who you are. Remember that **you are fearfully and wonderfully made, a marvelous creation indeed!** If you are such an extraordinary and wonderful creature, you absolutely must love yourself now, exactly as you are. Yes, I said now!

Do not wait until you weigh 10, 25 or 50 pounds less to make yourself beautiful or to love yourself.

How can you love others if you don't love yourself? You will tend to compare yourself and compete with others and/or become jealous of others. This is not what God desires. What He wants is for you to love yourself to such an extent that you can love others regardless of their shape and style. When we understand how God sees us, it changes all the misconceptions that the enemy has placed in our thoughts.

It's for one of those reasons I stopped looking at fashion magazines for a while. I always ended up comparing myself to women in those magazines and felt dissatisfied with myself. I was searching for the negative things in myself, and it made me lose sight of my goal.

Not Listening to Satan is a Choice

God wants us to love ourselves as He loves us. The Lord wants us to be proud of ourselves, that we see ourselves as marvelous creations. You should be proud of yourself today. Not listening to Satan's lies about you and hate yourself is a choice. You have the choice of loving yourself and maximizing your style and your potential.

Deep within yourself, your spirit knows that you are special. You are **unique** and no one can be who you are. Over time, I noticed that even the most marginal or different individuals who learned to love themselves became beautiful and remarkable people! If you focus on what complexes you, it will destroy and diminish what can emanate from you. However, if you focus right now on what you like and if you decide to love yourself, it will change your self-perception and the one others have of you.

Starting now, you must crave for more of yourself. Stop making comparisons between what others have and what you do not have. You have resources that God has given only to you and not to others. Be proud of who you are from now on. Become who you really are. Cherish your body, which is the temple of the Holy Spirit. Do not wait to be at your ideal weight to look your best. It is now and daily that you manifest the glory of God through you. Walk with your head held up high right now. Dress to look your best. Have the hairstyle

Cherish your body, which is the temple of the Holy Spirit.

you like. Wear make-up... **Most of all maximize who you are.** You are incomparable; you are unique! Every day, take care of yourself, feed your spirit, your soul and your body. These are essential gestures of self-esteem and self-love.

Your exterior reflects what goes on inside of you. If you fill your mind with the truth of God and the presence of the Holy Spirit, it will affect your soul and your body.

Find Your Passion

Your soul must be nourished by the truth. Your soul needs to be fulfilled. You must also be fulfilled. Find activities that stimulate you and make you feel good. Get moving! Do not stay without a passion. Find what you are passionate about and act on it. You will be motivated by what is in yourself and you will even forget at times to eat! For the time being, if you have no idea of what interests you, try different things. You will end up discovering your passion in life.

Get Moving!

Do not sit and do nothing, spending your evenings watching television. Get out... Go take a walk... Find an activity that interests you: tennis, physical training, swimming, bowling, skiing, skating, etc... Dance in your living room! Exercise! Activate your muscles... Enjoy yourself! I have seen too many people with weight problems who were passive and sedentary. Many were discouraged from doing physical activity because they were doing it only to lose weight and not to have fun in doing something good for them and take care of their body. Since your body is the temple of the Holy Spirit, get it moving to keep it in good shape. You must get moving in sports that you like. **If you do not like to move, do any physical activity, tell yourself that this resistance is still spiritual.** This spirit wants to prevent you from feeling good about yourself, putting all sorts of ideas in your mind to make you believe that you do not care much about exercising...

That is false! Humans were created to move, sweat, and be fulfilled... The muscles in your body want to be stronger. Your heart wants to be in shape... Your legs... Your arms... Get moving! Being on the move will do you good and you will quickly discover your body needs it. The enemy wants you to remain dejected, focusing on the negative side of things he has provoked so the heaviness settles and increases in your life. Quit this pattern immediately! Stop analyzing yourself in the mirror. Eliminate these obsessive thoughts planted by this spirit and do not stay inactive! Get out and move!

Remember that by applying the keys of this book, you will really be free and feel great about your body. It has nothing to do with what you eat or how long you do physical activity that will solve the problem, because the root of it is first of all spiritual. However, get active! As far as I was concerned, I was doing every possible effort to lose weight by dieting. I was training 4 to 5 days per week, but the results were only temporary...

Quality Sleep

Your body needs rest. Nothing beats a good sleep! It is proven that when a person does not have enough sleep, he or she will want to eat more to compensate for the lack of energy he feels. You must be disciplined regarding your hours of rest. The need to sleep is different for each person. Respect yours and you will see the difference. For my part, when I was lacking sleep, I felt more swollen. The enemy was using this against me to play with the perception I had of my body. I can tell you that realizing that has given me a weapon against these destructive thoughts: I made sure I went to bed earlier the following night.

Eating Well

Eating well is essential for our body to be well nourished and healthy. We must take care of the temple of the Holy Spirit, which is our body. I am against diets because it is frustrating control, without lasting results, just as eating poorly is. I still occasionally eat fast food, devoid of nourishment, but I don't consume it on a daily basis, knowing that such food is not what's best for my body. I love my body and I want to take good care of it. **I want to take good care of God's marvelous creation, what about you?** In doing so, we avoid feeling sick and forced to pray for physical healing because of our bad eating habits.

> *I love my body and I want to take good care of it.*

As a child of God, we must develop good eating habits and take care of our body, which is the temple of the Holy Spirit.

Throughout my spiritual journey, I discovered that the Holy Spirit was suggesting me and the right food to choose from. He knew exactly what my body needed. The more I obeyed what the Lord inspired me to eat, the better I felt in my body. I suggest you do the same thing. Your body requires specific things. Sometimes it needs more iron or vitamin C... Without your knowledge, you will find that by eating what the Lord inspires you to, you will feel filled and satisfied. Let the Holy Spirit be your guide!

Finally, it is also important to take good vitamin supplements to fill the void left by foods of poor quality. There is evidence to suggest that we can't find the same quality of nutrients in our food supply today than we did not so long ago. It is essential to choose healthy food for our body and add a good quality vitamin supplement because you know that our body is the temple of the Holy Spirit.

Be the head and not the tail; love and learn to appreciate yourself. Do not expect to be physically perfect before doing something. Many have a beautiful and healthy body, but they do not necessarily love themselves. Everything starts from within, and it starts right now!

3. Crave to Surround Yourself With People Who Crave For You

"When you surround yourself with loving mirrors, the world becomes a reflection of your true being and it is a beautiful vision."

In the past, I have long tried to be someone I was not so I could prove to others that I was worth something. If people did not give me the recognition I expected, it affected my self-esteem and the perception I had of myself. The more I persisted in this direction, the more I failed. I was more and more uncompromising towards myself; I was judging myself systematically and was consistently devaluing myself.

I Became a Product of My Surroundings...

At one point, I realized I was the product of my surroundings. I was not seeing myself as I should. Everything turned into negativity. The words received, the lack of encouragement and judgment crushed me. All the good that was within me was diluted. My perception was incorrect.

The day I started surrounding myself with rewarding, loving and comforting people, my self-image began to improve. As a matter of fact, one of the most significant persons in my life was my husband. He was the best gift I could have received at the time. I decided to love myself, recognize who I was, and crave for what was within me. Therefore, I could not continue to surround myself with indifferent or downright negative people.

The choice of my relationships was and continues to be important for Allen and I. You must now do the same thing. Surround yourself with positive people who respect you, raise you up, encourage you, believe in you and appreciate you. Do not waste your time with people who despise you, underestimate you, and to whom you must constantly prove yourself. Run in the other direction. You do not need that in your life. Even if you tried your hardest to change their perception of yourself and attitudes towards you, what would that give you? You must love your neighbor, but this does not mean to be close to him!

Surround yourself with people who honor you, not people who simply tolerate you. Go to those who crave for what is inside you. This will produce a positive impact on you and you will really feel like a marvelous creation of God! Make conscious efforts to surround yourself with positive, rewarding people who inspire you to be full of zeal and enthusiasm. People that believe in you, encourage you to realize your dreams, and achieve your goals, as well as capable of applauding your successes. These people will "pronounce words of life" over you to uplift your success and shine a light on your beauty. This will propel you to victory, which is to be free, and slim.

Count among your closest friends those whose life is an example, an inspiration. Try to have among your relationships people who are slim and free in their relationship with food. They can help you deprogram "viruses" regarding food and your body, and boost your self-esteem. Avoid people with low self-esteem, who will envy you when you begin to radiate more and more the glory of God.

> *Make conscious efforts to surround yourself with positive, rewarding people who inspire you to be full of zeal and enthusiasm. People that believe in you, encourage you to realize your dreams, and achieve your goals, as well as capable of applauding your successes.*

You Are the Temple of the Holy Spirit

Remind yourself that you are a royal priesthood, a holy people, a chosen race, the temple of the Holy Spirit, a creation of God that is so marvelous and a work that is so admirable. You must be ready to receive the best: the best creams, the most beautiful clothing and jewelry, the hairstyles that suit you the best... You are an ambassador, you represent the Kingdom of God and the best things in life must come to you.

People around you should respect you to the point where they see your potential and what is special in you.

Lift up your head! You're so important and special to God. Don't keep company with people who belittle you. The power of spiritual connection influences your life and your destiny. Connect yourself with people who will positively impact your life.

> *Remind yourself that you are a royal priesthood, a holy people, a chosen race, the temple of the Holy Spirit, a creation of God that's so marvelous and a work that's so admirable.*

Say This Prayer:

Lord,

On this day, I renounce the spirit of rejection, isolation, boredom and dependence on food.

I ask your forgiveness for having been dependent on food to meet the needs of my soul. On this day, I decide to be dependent on you alone.

I understand that you are my source, and it is you that meet all my needs and heal all my wounds from the past. Holy Spirit, fill me with your presence. Feed my soul with your unconditional love.

May my passion for you increase. May my craving for you intensify and may you fill all the voids within me. Thank you for changing my perception of myself and making me love myself as You love me. I pray that going forward, I may maximize my potential and that my life may glorify you.

Help me to take care of my body, which is your temple, and to feed it so it will be in excellent health.

Lord, that my personal relationships would improve by surrounding me with people who honor and encourage me, and who provide me with the enthusiasm needed for the realization of my dreams.

In the name of Jesus Christ. Amen!

Applying the Principles

- Everyday, ask God to live a passionate relationship with Him.

- Make a list of qualities you love about yourself (personality, gifts, physical...). Stick this "for your eyes only" list in a place where you will see it frequently, such as your wardrobe. Read it DAY AFTER DAY, thanking the Lord for the wonderful creature you are.

- Crave to be fulfilled. Find activities you enjoy and be creative...

- Move! Make one or more physical activities that you enjoy.

- Cherish yourself through the choices you make towards food, exercise and the clothes you wear.

- Consume good quality vitamins to compensate for deficiencies in the food you eat.

- Sleep well. If you have trouble sleeping, this problem must be solved with the Lord's help.

- Surround yourself with people who are craving for you, what is inside you; people who raise you up, honor you and applaud your successes.

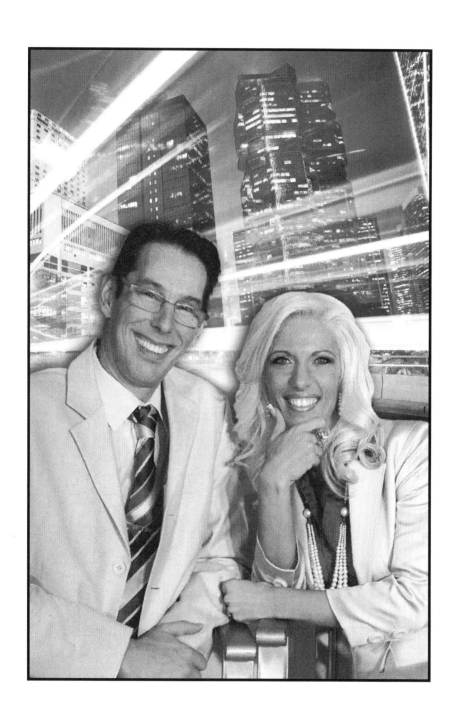

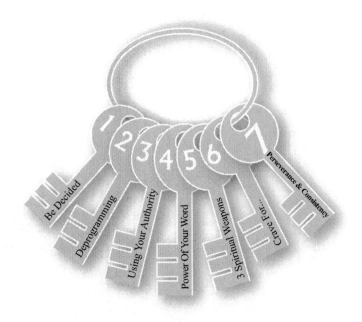

PERSEVERANCE AND CONSISTENCY

"Winners never quit and quitters never win."

PERSEVERANCE AND CONSISTENCY

his is the last key that's just as important as the other six. In fact, the first key and the latter accompany all the others. **You absolutely need this last one to obtain absolute victory over food and with your body.** It allows you to reach the desired result and keep it. Remain consistent in your decision.

By observing successful people, I discovered that it was not where they came from that mattered, but rather where they were finally going. As we have seen in previous chapters, all of us have not grown in the same soil. Some have grown in a harsher soil with many nutritional deficiencies, while others have developed in richer, more fertile soils. However, God enjoys taking what looked completely destroyed and turning it into a vessel of honor. Keep your eyes fixed on the promises of God for your life; promises of freedom, peace, health, and wellbeing.

I grew up in a Christian family and I was surrounded all my life with Christians. **I can tell you that as children of God, we must learn to be more perseverant and consistent.** I saw so many people excited to the extreme by a new project, and eventually abandoning it. I am not saying you should not be excited, but I want you to understand that we must remain passionate and constant, even if some days, the enemy tries to slow us down with his strategies.

After reading this book, remember that the first strategies Satan will use against you will be to make you lose your enthusiasm and to distract you. He knows that you are the only person who can stop the blessing of God.

> *"That ye be not slothful, but followers of them who through **faith and patience** inherit the promises."*
>
> *Hebrews 6:12*

We must have faith, patience and perseverance to obtain our promises. We see that in many biblical stories; that perseverance, determination, and persistence led to wars and revolutions being won throughout history.

Nehemiah

Nehemiah was a man of God from the Old Testament. His story touched

He never quit.

me deeply these past few years. I learned a lot through this man's attitude. After learning the walls of Jerusalem had been destroyed, Nehemiah had in his heart to rebuild the city and bring it up from destruction. This man was determined to bring about the vision he had received in his heart from start to finish. Despite the enemy's attacks, treason and sometimes lack of support, he never quit. Ever! He persevered and day after day, put strategies in place to defeat the conniving plans of the enemy. Finally, Nehemiah could celebrate his victory and go rest peacefully because he had fulfilled the vision in his heart.

It's the same for you... What is on your heart – to be completely free and slender – will be perfectly and completely fulfilled, if you never cease to persevere. Despite the days when you feel the enemy prowling around and putting all sorts of thoughts in your head, playing with your emotions, **you will not quit**. You know it is only a tactic of Satan to stop and steal your rewards. So, you will continue to focus on the same goal, keep the vision fresh in your mind and implement the **777 Program** every day to go from glory to glory!

Noah

> *Noah decided to trust God's Word.*

The story of Noah shows this man of God decided to obey the Word of God rather than trust in human thought. He began to build a ship, an ark, despite the fact that it had never rained on earth before. Imagine that! The wisdom of God is foolishness to man. You know the rest of the story: one day, the rain came and no one expected it, but Noah was saved and blessed! How much this story is valuable to realize that Noah decided to trust God's Word. He knew it would be accomplished and he inherited the promise to see his family saved! **Everyone else died because they refused to believe in the Word of God. They preferred to listen to the wisdom of the majority of the people.**

On whose side do you want to be? On the side of God's wisdom and what His Word says, or the side of human wisdom and what people say on TV, your family, your spouse, and your friends if they are not saved?

Noah decided to only listen to the Word of God, to put his trust in it, and persevere until the rain came. And that is exactly what happened! In deciding to keep your eyes on God and His wisdom, and to relentlessly persevere, you will see, like Noah, God's promise come true in your life; which is to be free to eat what you want and remain slim!

David

> *He was not perfect, he made mistakes, but he never quit.*

Here is another man of God who persevered and inherited the promises of the Lord. As you can see in David's story, **he has been through many obstacles, but came out winning**. From the day he was anointed by the prophet Samuel to become king, to the day he was acclaimed king, he had to fight both spiritually and physically. If David had quit, he could have never entered into the promises God had in store for him.

Satan knew David's heart, and he absolutely wanted to stop God's plan in his life. He knew the impact David would have on all the people as king. David decided to keep his eyes on God's promises and refused to rely on circumstances and desperate situations. He was not perfect, he made mistakes, but he never quit. He kept faith in God. He spoke to his own soul and refused to enter Satan's playground with fear. He enjoyed victory after victory.

234

"Now faith is the substance of things hoped for, the evidence of things not seen."

Hebrews 11:1

Do as David: Keep your eyes focused on fighting the good fight! Have faith that God will accomplish what He has promised you. Be firm in your hope in God's Word. Be a warrior like David to win your case. By persevering like him, you will glorify God through your life and have a significant impact on the lives of others.

Daniel

Daniel is a concrete example of determination and perseverance. When he was brought to King Nebuchadnezzar as a prisoner, he refused to comply with everyone else's way of eating in the kingdom and decided to continue to pray his God, despite the king's opposition and official decree. He persisted to think and act according to God's principles. **He didn't listen to man, but to the voice of the Holy Spirit, and he was greatly blessed.**

As a child of God, the example to follow is exactly the same. Are you more influenced by the mentality of man or God? Are you influenced by someone appearing to be wise

Are you more influenced by the mentality of man or God? Who do you listen to the most? The world or God?

according to the world's standards, and do you espouse his or her philosophy? Who do you listen to the most? The world or God? With all the teachings of truth you received in this book, you can fully turn to God and say: "Lord, I believe and I live according to Your Word, and not to the thought of men."

Esther

Her determination and faith in God enabled her to achieve victory.

When I was young, the story of Esther was the one I preferred. I admired the courage and determination of this woman of God. It remains true today. Her story tells of her position as a Jewish woman who became queen and wife of the Babylonian King Ahasuerus. After an edict put forth by him to kill all Jews, Esther had to find strategies to save her people. She ordered a three-day fast for everybody and prayed to God to reveal to her the strategies and actions to defeat the enemy's plans. This woman of God defied the law, stating that she deserved death if she appeared before the king without his permission and strategically managed to save her people.

Her determination and faith in God enabled her to achieve victory. It's exactly the same thing for you today. Faith in your God and His Word, couple with your determination to be free and slim; will propel you towards the destiny God has for you, marvelous creation of God!

236

And Several Others...

The Bible contains several stories that demonstrate perseverance, consistency, and determination. We also see it with Abraham, Joseph, Moses, Joshua, Rahab, Naomi & Ruth, Solomon, Elijah, Elisha, Anna, Paul, Peter, and John... They are men and women of God who conquered by their faith and perseverance. Hallelujah! You are now the generation that can show the world that even in this area of your life, which is to be free and slim, you can get your promises, and glorify the name of God.

> *"He also that is slothful in his work is brother to him that is a great waster."*
>
> *Proverbs 18:9*

Achieving true freedom and true slenderness is a process that cannot be completed in 24 hours. It starts now and gradually develops until you reach your objectives.

The lack of persistence and perseverance is the lot of all losers. They have slackened, which led them to their destruction. **In the 777 Program, it's absolutely out of the question to act in this manner!** It is a new programming as a new attitude for the rest of your life. Achieving true freedom and true slenderness is a process that cannot be completed in 24 hours. It starts now and gradually develops. A certain amount of time is needed to cleanse your soul and realign your body without deprivation. The final key to obtain your promises is unmistakably persistence and consistency!

> *"But he **who** looks carefully into the faultless law, the [law] of liberty, and is faithful to it and **perseveres** in looking into it, being not a heedless listener who forgets but an active doer [who obeys], he **shall be blessed** in his doing (his life of obedience)."*
>
> James 1:25 *(Amplified Bible)*

Persevere!

Understand that the word persevere in this verse means:
- Adhere to…
- Dedication to...
- Keep one's attention fixed on...
- Focus on...
- Always carry on in the same direction
- Be brave
- Be rigorous amid your constancy
- Be patient in action

In the Oxford dictionary, the word "perseverance" is defined as a steady persistence in adhering to a course of action, a belief, or a purpose; steadfastness. Remain firm and consistent in a decision, or the action taken. Moreover, the word "consistency" is defined as the moral strength of a person who doesn't let anything discourage him or her. **Let's realize the importance of these qualities on our determination... In James 1:25, God teaches us the need to carry on in the same direction, be courageous, thorough, stand firm, and not be daunted by anything to be blessed and inherit our promises.** Did you know that this 7th key is the one that accompanies the 6 previous keys, giving them power to propel you toward freedom and slenderness?

You Must Be Perseverant and Consistent:

1. In your decision to be free and slim.

2. In deprogramming viruses and reprogramming your mind according to the Word of God.

3. In using your divine authority.

4. In the way you talk about food and your body.

5. In fasting, sowing and praying.

6. In your craving for God, for yourself and by surrounding yourself of people who crave for you.

7. And finally, in applying the 777 Program, day after day, week after week.

Falling Is Not Failing, Not Getting Up Is

It is impossible to think that we will never fall. Some days are more difficult than others, and Satan comes to attack us in the moments we are more vulnerable and tired. However, the Word of God is clear regarding these days of resistance.

"For a just man falleth seven times, and riseth up again."

Proverbs 24:16 a

What God is telling us is that the just falls, but he has the strength to get up and continue. What is within him is stronger than the attack of the enemy. He does not stay down, but stands up again. He perseveres, is constant, determined, tenacious, and does not let himself be beaten down.

Satan Is the Accuser

If you get up, you will win!

Satan enjoys making the just fall. He whispers to his ears that he is nothing, that he is defeated and that finally he will never accomplish something good in life. In this area of his life, which is to be free and slim, he will never be victorious. Satan is a liar! He wants to throw you down and then accuse you that it is your fault and that you will stay down. Throughout the years, I realized the important thing is to pick yourself up. If you do, you will win, this is guaranteed! It is not the number of times you fall that matters, but that each time you do fall, you get up and persevere.

Do you believe those who are successful have never fallen? On the contrary, if you read their biographies, all those who made history have fallen several times in their lives. However, they never lost their objectives and persevered until they achieved their goals. They have not kept their focus on what made them fall, but on the goals and strategies they put in place to achieve success.

> *They have not kept their focus on what made them fall, but on the goals and strategies they put in place to achieve success.*

Your Attitude Determines Your Altitude

It is a spiritual law God created. He left us free to choose for ourselves. If you choose to win and persevere, something will happen... Your victory! **Never believe that others are born to be free with regards to food and slim, and that God has isolated you from this blessing and deprived you of it in your life. Wrong! Perseverance and consistency in implementing the 777 Program will bring this absolute victory in your life too.** As long as you do not quit, you will not lose. Keep your eyes on the goal. The only reason why people fail is they cease to persevere, and therefore, they don't reach their goal. They get distracted, look back, still seeing only their failures and forgetting to persevere everyday so they can reach the promised land.

You are among those who hold on and stand firm. Tell yourself that no matter how long it will take, only results matter. This promise to be slim and free is for you. **Persevere with faith and patience and you will have your victory!**

The only reason why people fail is they cease to persevere, and therefore, they don't reach their goal.

Say This Prayer:

Lord Jesus,

Thank you for all the revelations I received in this book and thank you for helping me implement them in my life.

By your all-powerful strength, I will not lose sight of my goal, I will persevere and be persistent to obtain my promises.

All past failures are over, and I have the assurance and certainty I will be victorious. I'm determined to persevere. I have the firm assurance that I will see my victory in the natural, because I will persevere until I achieve complete victory over food and my weight issues.

I glorify You for what You have done so far in my life, and what You will do for me in the coming weeks.

In the name of Jesus Christ. Amen!

Applying the Principles

- Be perseverent and consistent in using your authority as a child of God.

- Use perseverence and consistency in the way you talk about food and your body.

- Persevere and be consistent in fasting (3 days x 7 weeks or 21 consecutive days), in sowing (the exact amount and place God puts in your heart) and in prayer.

- You must persevere and be consistent in your craving for God, yourself, as well as surrounding yourself with people who crave for you.

- And finally, be perseverent and consistent in applying this 777 Program day after day, week after week.

- Repeat the 777 Program until you reach your goals.

- Persevere to think as God thinks, and not as men do.

- Persevere always. If some days are harder, if you fall... Pick yourself up and go on!

- Remember that this key is as important as the other six.

- You must be perseverent and consistent in your decision to be free and slim.

- You must also be perseverent and consistent in the deprogramming of "viruses" and reprogramming according to the Word of God.

Conclusion

You are a part of the Army of God and with this book in your hands, you have all the tools needed for victory. And what a victory! God has no limits... With God, anything is possible, even when everything seems impossible. You have a God of action! If you implement His operating system and act according to the spiritual laws He created, your success will be your result. The application of this 7 key program over 7 weeks for freedom in your relationship with food and slenderness will help you to understand and apply the powerful lessons that you've received.

Do Not Let Go! If You Fall... Pick Yourself Up!

You now know that it is not falling that matters, but actually getting up again. I am living proof that God's system works... And I'm not alone! The testimonies in this book also confirm it. God can make you free and slim. If you applied the principles, you are already seeing the changes of a major transformation. Stop the wrong programming received in your life and that perhaps, you are still getting. Do not utter negative words over yourself, things like: "I am fat, I will always have cellulite, varicose veins, etc." Do not accept the destructive words of others about yourself either. A negative thought can be repeated up to 600 times a day. It is time to pick yourself up, see victory and proclaim your slenderness through your mouth! Adopt God's system as your new lifestyle. God's promises do not stop after reading the book. Beware of Satan, this prowling liar and thief. He only waits for the moment when he can steal your success. You received this book to get out of his pitfalls and tactics aimed at intimidating and destroying you.

As a Child of God, Be Decided to Go From Glory to Glory!

Keep this book close at hand at all times to thwart the plans of the enemy. I encourage you to look in a mirror and speak the truth of God on yourself, on your body. Pray as often as possible. What comes out of your mouth is powerful and can effectively combat the devil and his kingdom. The victory is yours! Review the root(s) of the problem... You will certainly find other points to correct along the way, and they will give you even more altitude. You know the old saying: your attitude determines your altitude!

The more you read and reread this book, the more you become victorious with God's truth, which shall make you free. All its content is worthy of all your attention. **Even when we think we have absorbed the teachings, we discover a new principle or a small thing that makes all the difference and helps us go even further!** The 7 keys are miraculous for those who implement them. What you believe is what you receive. We need only one revelation to eradicate the lies of the enemy... You have received several! Consciously apply these teachings by taking 7 minutes per day and practicing only 1 key per week for the next 7 weeks. You'll see the power of the 777 Program in your soul and in your body.

246

Remember that God's Word is The Truth! You are made in the image of God. Keep your mouth under control. Speak to your soul at all times! Decree who you really are! Prophesy everything that's good over your body and your life! If your slenderness is not yet visible in the natural realm, it is already accomplished in the spiritual one. It is time to take ownership of your body and freedom in your relationship with food. Say right now: "I am slim... I choose to be FREE AND SLIM." HALLELUJAH!

GOD'S TRUTH IS ALWAYS TRIUMPHANT!

I pray for all the readers of this book to be touched and transformed by the truth, the Word of God and the anointing. I keep you in my prayers for your total victory!

With All My Love,

Martine Wilkie

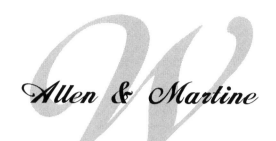

Ministères **Wilkie** Ministries

To learn more about
Wilkie Ministries, write to us at:

Wilkie Ministries

600, rue Pierre-Caisse, C.P. 40013

St-Jean-sur-Richelieu, Quebec, Canada

J3A 1L0

Contact us at:
ministries@wilkieminitries.com

Visit our website:

www.AllenMartine.tv

Appendices

APPENDIX 1

Testimonies

MRS. JEANNE TREMBLAY

I would like to thank Pastor Martine for this extraordinary opportunity I had to experience "Be Free, Be Slim" in a group setting. Everything starts with a decision to begin something with perseverance. What got me hooked right from the start is above all the word "free" in the title of the course. What I wanted to achieve by following this course was to feel good about myself. There were many things I dragged behind me and I knew that through this course I would be made free. First, I would like to thank God, for I am now healed of diabetes. Hallelujah! That is what I asked for initially. I also learned to listen to my body, to eat less and eat more slowly. I realized that we are not obligated to eat three meals a day, as we were taught to do. I learned to listen to my body's needs and talk to it: "Am I hungry? Am I thirsty? Etc."

In my childhood I heard my father say: "My tall ugly girl! My tall unattractive girl!" Consequently, I never found myself beautiful. I was afraid of growing old and I asked the Lord to deliver me from my fears. I broke these negative words by the authority that I received as a child of God. My husband helped me a lot as well. Since these teachings, he decrees daily on me that I am more and more beautiful, and I am pleased with myself now. It is wonderful to get up in the morning and look in the mirror and say, "Thank you Lord, I am fearfully and wonderfully made, a marvelous creation!" I am approaching my sixties now, and I cannot believe my age. I'm pleased to be where I am now, and this course gave me the strength and perseverance to get there. The first key, "The Power of Decision," allowed me to take action and decide that everything that had been programmed in my childhood was over. Today, I begin a new life at age 60. Even if sometimes we feel like letting go, we persevere; thanks to the tangible results we have received. I think about my husband, Michel Gagnon, this new man, 55 pounds (25 kg) lighter. He can also claim to have a new woman in his life. The Word of God through the power of our words has transformed us. The past is behind us. We are moving toward the future with a new lifestyle. My husband and I apply the 7 keys we learned in the "Be Free, Be Slim" course in every area of our lives. It is not over... This is just the beginning! We go from glory to glory together!

Jeanne Tremblay
St-Jean-sur-Richelieu, Quebec, Canada

Mr. Eric Beaulieu

I've been with the Wilkie Ministries for several years now. When Pastor Martine decided to offer the "Be Free, Be Slim" course, I was invited to offer technical assistance for it. I also had in my heart to be there to learn, remember and apply these principles.

I didn't have much weight to lose. I did a lot of sports in my life, but when my children were born, I stopped. However, I continued to eat the same way. Therefore, I gradually accumulated some unsightly bulges that I wanted to see disappear.

During each week of the course when we talked about the different keys like prayer, the power of our words, fasting, etc., I knew these keys were very important. Something touched me deeply: the realization **that gluttony is a sin**. When Pastor Martine talked about it, it was as though the Holy Spirit had pointed the finger at me and spoken to my soul: "Look Eric, gluttony is a sin. If you want to please me, you must stop overeating. In this area too, you must walk according to my Word."

I am from the Saguenay-Lac Saint-Jean region, and we enjoy eating in this part of the country. Each meal always ends with dessert, even if we're more or less hungry. These are bad habits for the body that can only serve to accumulate fat. You feel less free indeed when you are overweight.

Right at the beginning of the course, I decided to closely monitor my diet. I always asked myself questions about whether or not I was hungry for a second serving, if the chocolate bar as a snack or the bag of potato chips in the evening was really necessary, etc.

By putting into practice, with my wife, the keys that we had received, I realized that God had intervened on my body and I was supernaturally losing weight. At the beginning of the course, I weighed 196 pounds (89 kg), and at the end of the implementation of the 777 Program, I had already lost a little over 11 pounds (5 kg). My wife and I continued to speak words of life on ourselves and keep the new dietary habits we had developed. We also fasted for 21 days to get answers in different areas of our lives. Following the different steps we took with determination, we received the answers we were seeking. I've now lost 24 pounds (11 kg) and I feel great in my body and free to eat what I want when I'm hungry.

I would like to warmly thank Pastor Martine for sharing these teachings. I sincerely believe that if people decide to carefully read this book and totally get involved with the goal to implement the principles, their life and their eating habits will completely change. They will also feel free in this area of their lives and, if they so desire, in other areas as well, since the keys shared here can be useful at so many other levels.

Congratulations for your book! It includes invaluable keys. All those who will put its content into practice will witness miracles and see their lives completely changed. May the Lord richly bless them!

Eric Beaulieu
Saint-Basile-le-Grand, Quebec, Canada

Mrs. Chantal Frégeau

I used to feel good in my body and my soul. I am not someone who nibbles or eats poorly. However, in the past two years, my thoughts and my body began to change. When I sat down to eat, I found everything so tasty that I did not feel like stopping to eat and went over the limits of my appetite. A spirit of gluttony was slowly creeping in. I thought it was not so bad if I went over my limit; I was to eat less at the next meal, which I ultimately never did.

Being in my forties, there was also a lie that I had started to believe, that I was bound to gain weight, that I was going to have the thighs about which my mother complained, that I would find myself gaining weight as a result of menopause. So there was the fear of gaining weight, a certain fear of aging and over time, I was enjoying myself physically less and less.

Through the "Be Free, Be Slim" course, I became able to understand that I did not need to accept these lies. I learned about what was coming against my body and me: I do not accept feeling plump or bloated anymore; I do not want anymore recurring negative thoughts in my spirit. I learned that gluttony was a sin, that we must bring this overeating before God, who gave food for the belly, not the other way around, the belly for food. I understood how our body showed it had a curse through being overweight or worse still, developing a disease! Therefore, we are not free in our minds anymore.

By proclaiming beautiful words of life during these several weeks of classes, I felt like running towards the freedom that God promised me. Promises of health, peace, happiness and well-being, and how important it is to keep them. I realized even more how God loved us, how we are precious in His eyes, how He wants to take care of us. Therefore, this was reflected in all areas of my life. Moreover, I realized how I had authority over the things that concerned me. I wanted to fast even more to come against the enemy and proclaim words of life concerning everything in my life. I put a distance between food and myself: after all, food only serves to meet our physical needs. I remain alert to make sure the spirit of gluttony has no more influence on me by asking myself if I am still hungry.

I lost 11 pounds (7 kg) and must confess that after the 21-day fast with my husband, I felt marvelously well! God took care of all my needs. I recommend it to everyone. I feel I am in a transformation process. Through certain divine revelations, ties have been broken and this is only the beginning!

Thank you Pastor Martine for these revelations that bring about changes we can see today, and for the rest of our lives!

Chantal Frégeau
Saint-Basile-le-Grand, Quebec, Canada

Mrs. Véronique Naurais

Allen and Martine's ministry has changed my life. It had a powerful impact on my life, since I made a complete about face: I decided to give up witchcraft. I worked in the astrology field for the past 20 years.

The "Be Free, Be Slim" course was a very important trigger. Through these weekly meetings, I received a special anointing of teachings that cannot be found anywhere else. I realized which difficulties or obstacles were blocking my success. Among other things, when they talked about generational ties, I recognized that the familiar spirit of witchcraft came from my family and that in order to live in the light and become slimmer, I had to begin by breaking this tie.

Similarly, as far as my education was concerned, I had to deprogram lies that I had come to believe, such as: "You don't eat enough ... You'll be sick!" Unlike the rest of my family, I did not eat the same way as them and often, my parents had to force me to eat. In my early childhood, they even hired someone to make me eat, because I could spend many hours chewing the same mouthful. I was often criticized for snacking. For me personally, I had to overcome the sixth root: Fear. Relatives often entertained certain fears on my sister and myself. I had to take authority over all this in order to get rid of it and start losing weight.

The power of our words is important and as a writer, I always paid attention to the words I used. Since the teaching of the key "The Power of the Words", I watch everything I say. I know it makes a difference for my family and me. Having been through a surgery to remove both of my ovaries and quitting smoking at the same time, like many people, I was conditioning myself that I would gain weight. I am currently about to deprogram myself from all this. Thanks to the "Be Free, Be Slim" course, I started losing weight.

However, the real trigger that made a difference is when I decided to leave the world of darkness by not practicing astrology and to enter into the Kingdom of God. The power of my words helped me, coupled with fasting and sowing. Do not overlook these since we offer them directly to God. Many requests were answered and generational ties were broken through these three powerful weapons. I thank God for having directed Pastors Martine and Allen on my path. Glory to God!

Véronique Naurais
Mont-Saint-Hilaire, Quebec, Canada

MRS. CAROLINE LECLERC

I give glory to God for what He has done in my life and what He continues to do. I thank Pastor Martine for her obedience to Him in sharing with others the revelations she received. Since I've started using the 7 keys and applying the 777 Program, my life has changed considerably. My relationship with food has changed. I lost weight and continue to lose weight. Since then, I have completely revamped my closet three times!

Previously, I ate until I was badly bloated and forced to undo the button of my pants. I dieted so often that I can't count the number of times I decided to start a new diet on Monday morning! My first diets date back to my teenage years. This problem is generational. Now that the 777 Program has become a lifestyle, my life has completely changed.

Before eating, during and towards the end of the meal, I ask myself questions such as: "Am I hungry or thirsty?", "Am I still hungry?", "Am I still hungry or is it simply a meal I like so much that I would want to lick the plate?", "Will I finish my meal in the restaurant, although I'm not hungry, because it's more expensive?"

I discovered that I didn't drink enough throughout the day. You know, when you have gone through so many diets, there are certain foods that you're no longer able to consume. For my part, I had trouble drinking water, but now that I'm

260

FREE, I drink a lot of it and I do not feel obligated to do so. I drink because I am thirsty! I discovered that sometimes I drink more than I eat, and my body does not complain about it.

Fasting has really been a revelation for me. I do not fast to lose weight, but to get closer to God, and my body benefits from it at the same time.

With "Be Free, Be Slim", the program that Pastor Martine implemented by the revelations given to her by God, I have a better self-esteem now. I regularly speak words of life about myself; what God says about me, not what people in the world are saying. I am a marvelous creation of God, and everyone around me could testify I am truly melting away and that I am more beautiful day after day! My life goes from glory to glory! I thank you Lord for having transformed me. I recommend this book to anyone who is really determined to see changes in this area of their lives and I know from my experience, that when you feel good about yourself and your body, you are happier. Self-esteem is restored with these teachings. We are ready for anything, but we must really be determined and persevere.

Caroline Leclerc
St-Jean-sur-Richelieu, Quebec, Canada

Appendix 2

A Few Verses

"We will rejoice in thy salvation, and in the name of our God we will set up our banners: the Lord fulfill all thy petitions. Now know I that the Lord saveth his anointed; he will hear him from his holy heaven with the saving strength of his right hand."

Psalms 20:5- 6

"Blessed be the Lord, because he hath heard the voice of my supplications. The Lord is my strength and my shield; my heart trusted in him, and I am helped: therefore my heart greatly rejoiceth; and with my song will I praise him."

Psalms 28:6- 7

"Our soul waiteth for the Lord: he is our help and our shield."

Psalms 33:20

"Keep thy tongue from evil, and thy lips from speaking guile."

Psalms 34:13

262

"Many are the afflictions of the righteous: but the Lord delivereth him out of them all."

Psalms 34:19

"Delight thyself also in the Lord: and he shall give thee the desires of thine heart."

Psalms 37:4

"For I will not trust in my bow, neither shall my sword save me. But thou hast saved us from our enemies, and hast put them to shame that hated us. In God we boast all the day long, and praise thy name for ever. Selah. But thou hast cast off, and put us to shame; and goest not forth with our armies."

Psalms 44:6- 9

"Thou wilt prolong the king's life: and his years as many generations."

Psalms 61:6

"He only is my rock and my salvation: he is my defence; I shall not be moved."

Psalms 62:6

"For thou hast possessed my reins: thou hast covered me in my mother's womb. I will praise thee; for I am fearfully and wonderfully made: marvellous are thy works; and that my soul knoweth right well. My substance was not hid from thee, when I was made in secret, and curiously wrought in the lowest parts of the earth. Thine eyes did see my substance, yet being unperfect; and in thy book all my members were written, which in continuance were fashioned, when as yet there was none of them."

Psalms 139:13- 16

"Thou art snared with the words of thy mouth, thou art taken with the words of thy mouth."

Proverbs 6:2

"He that keepeth his mouth keepeth his life: but he that openeth wide his lips shall have destruction."

Proverbs 13:3

"The heart of the wise teacheth his mouth, and addeth learning to his lips. Pleasant words are as an honeycomb, sweet to the soul, and health to the bones."

Proverbs 16:23-24

"A man's belly shall be satisfied with the fruit of his mouth; and with the increase of his lips shall he be filled. Death and life are in the power of the tongue: and they that love it shall eat the fruit thereof."

Proverbs 18:20- 21

"Whoso keepeth his mouth and his tongue keepeth his soul from troubles."

Proverbs 21:23

"Thou art all fair, my love; there is no spot in thee."

Song of Songs 4:7

"Is not this the fast that I have chosen? to loose the bands of wickedness, to undo the heavy burdens, and to let the oppressed go free, and that ye break every yoke? Is it not to deal thy bread to the hungry, and that thou bring the poor that are cast out to thy house? when thou seest the naked, that thou cover him; and that thou hide not thyself from thine own flesh? Then shall thy light break forth as the morning, and thine health shall spring forth speedily: and thy righteousness shall go before thee; the glory of the Lord shall be thy rearward. Then shalt thou call, and the Lord shall answer; thou shalt cry, and he shall say, Here I am. If thou take away from the midst of thee the yoke, the putting forth of the finger, and speaking vanity; And if thou draw out thy soul to the hungry, and satisfy the afflicted soul; then shall thy light rise in obscurity, and thy darkness be as the noon day: And the Lord shall guide thee continually, and satisfy thy soul in drought, and make fat thy bones: and thou shalt be like a watered garden, and like a spring of water, whose waters fail not. And they that shall be of thee shall build the old waste places: thou shalt raise up the foundations of many generations; and thou shalt be called, The repairer of the breach, The restorer of paths to dwell in. If thou turn away thy foot from the sabbath, from doing thy

pleasure on my holy day; and call the sabbath a delight, the holy of the Lord, honourable; and shalt honour him, not doing thine own ways, nor finding thine own pleasure, nor speaking thine own words: Then shalt thou delight thyself in the Lord; and I will cause thee to ride upon the high places of the earth, and feed thee with the heritage of Jacob thy father: for the mouth of the Lord hath spoken it."

(Fasting) Isaiah 58:6-14

"And therefore will the Lord wait, that he may be gracious unto you, and therefore will he be exalted, that he may have mercy upon you: for the Lord is a God of judgment: blessed are all they that wait for him!"

Isaiah 30:18

"Surely he hath borne our griefs, and carried our sorrows: yet we did esteem him stricken, smitten of God, and afflicted. But he was wounded for our transgressions, he was bruised for our iniquities: the chastisement of our peace was upon him; and with his stripes we are healed."

Isaiah 53:4- 5

"The Spirit of the Lord God is upon me; because the Lord hath anointed me to preach good tidings unto the meek; he hath sent me to bind up the brokenhearted, to proclaim liberty to the captives, and the opening of the prison to them that are bound; To proclaim the acceptable year of the Lord, and the day of vengeance of our God; to comfort all that mourn; To appoint unto them that mourn in Zion, to give unto them beauty for ashes, the oil of joy for mourning, the garment of praise for the spirit of heaviness; that they might be called trees of righteousness, the planting of the Lord, that he might be glorified."

Isaiah 61: 1- 3

"My people are destroyed for lack of knowledge: because thou hast rejected knowledge, I will also reject thee, that thou shalt be no priest to me: seeing thou hast forgotten the law of thy God, I will also forget thy children."

Hosea 4:6

"Blessed are they that mourn: for they shall be comforted!"

Matthew 5:4

268

"If ye then, being evil, know how to give good gifts unto your children, how much more shall your Father which is in heaven give good things to them that ask him?"

Matthew 7:11

"And Jesus saith unto him, I will come and heal him."

Matthew 8:7

"O generation of vipers, how can ye, being evil, speak good things? For out of the abundance of the heart the mouth speaketh."

Matthew 12:34

"For verily I say unto you, That whosoever shall say unto this mountain, Be thou removed, and be thou cast into the sea; and shall not doubt in his heart, but shall believe that those things which he saith shall come to pass; he shall have whatsoever he saith."

Mark 11:23

"And take heed to yourselves, lest at any time your hearts be overcharged with surfeiting, and drunkenness, and cares of this life, and so that day come upon you unawares."

Luke 21:34

"Let us walk honestly, as in the day; not in rioting and drunkenness, not in chambering and wantonness, not in strife and envying."

Romans 13:13

"If any man defile the temple of God, him shall God destroy; for the temple of God is holy, which temple ye are."

1 Corinthians 3:17

"All things are lawful unto me, but all things are not expedient: all things are lawful for me, but I will not be brought under the power of any. Meats for the belly, and the belly for meats: but God shall destroy both it and them. Now the body is not for fornication, but for the Lord; and the Lord for the body."

1 Corinthians 6:12-13

"For though we walk in the flesh, we do not war after the flesh: For the weapons of our warfare are not carnal, but mighty through God to the pulling down of strong holds."

2 Corinthians 10:3- 4

"Christ hath redeemed us from the curse of the law, being made a curse for us: for it is written, Cursed is every one that hangeth on a tree."

Galatians 3:13

270

"And if ye be Christ's, then are ye Abraham's seed, and heirs according to the promise."

Galatians 3:29

"Now the works of the flesh are manifest, which are these; Adultery, fornication, uncleanness, lasciviousness. Idolatry, witchcraft, hatred, variance, emulations, wrath, strife, seditions, heresies. Envyings, murders, drunkenness, revellings, and such like: of the which I tell you before, as I have also told you in time past, that they which do such things shall not inherit the kingdom of God"

(Gluttony) Galatians 5:19- 21

"Wherefore take unto you the whole armor of God, that ye may be able to withstand in the evil day, and having done all, to stand."

Ephesians 6:13

"For God hath not given us the spirit of fear; but of power, and of love, and of a sound mind."

2 Timothy 1:7

"That ye be not slothful, but followers of them who through faith and patience inherit the promises."

Hebrews 6:12

"Now faith is the substance of things hoped for, the evidence of things not seen."

Hebrews 11:1

"Through faith we understand that the worlds were framed by the word of God, so that things which are seen were not made of things which do appear."

Hebrew 11:3

"Wherefore lift up the hands which hang down, and the feeble knees; And make straight paths for your feet, lest that which is lame be turned out of the way; but let it rather be heale."

Hebrews 12:12- 13

"For the time past of our life may suffice us to have wrought the will of the Gentiles, when we walked in lasciviousness, lusts, excess of wine, revellings, banquetings, and abominable idolatries."

1 Peter 4:3

"While they promise them liberty, they themselves are the servants of corruption: for of whom a man is overcome, of the same is he brought in bondage."

2 Peter 2:19

"For the truth's sake, which dwelleth in us, and shall be with us for ever."

3 John 1:2

THE PRAYER OF REPENTANCE

Prayer to receive Christ in your life

At this moment you can pronounce the most important prayer of your life by saying:

Lord Jesus,

I believe that You are the Son of God. I believe that You came on earth 2,000 years ago. I believe that You died on the cross for me and that you shed Your blood for my Salvation. I believe that You rose from the dead and went up to heaven. I believe that You will come back on earth.

Dear Jesus, I am a sinner. Forgive my sins. Purify me now with Your precious blood. Come in my heart. Save my soul now. I give you my life. I receive You as my Savior, my Lord and my God. I belong to You forever. I will serve You and follow You for the rest of my life. From now on I belong to You. I no longer belong to this world. I am now born again.

Amen!

By saying this prayer to receive Jesus Christ in your heart and by confessing your sins, God has given the right to become His child.

> *"But as many as received him, to then he gave the poser to become the sons of God, even to them that believe on his name."*
>
> *John 1:12*

You just received Jesus Christ in your life;
we want to rejoice with you!

Share it with us:

www.AllenMartine.tv

777 Program

Be determined and...
Persevere for an
absolute victory!

- Apply the 777 Program:
  7 keys, 7 minutes a day during 7 weeks

- Use the application grids offered

- Take 7 minutes each day to assimilate the key
  that corresponds with the week where you are
  and keep the previous ones.

- Say also the prayers and apply the required
  principles

7 keys
for an absolute victory
over food and
your body

1ˢᵗ WEEK - DATE: _____

THE POWER OF DECISION

Applying the Principles

Done

- Take time to understand the previous lessons to obtain a complete divine victory. ☐

- Be determined to face the root(s) of the problem you have identified in the second chapter. This is important! ☐

- Close the door to all your fears in the name of Jesus Christ. No demon can stop you if you are determined. ☐

- Be determined to take authority over what comes against you and to reprogram yourself according to the Word of God. ☐

- Do not deprive yourself. Frustration and deprivation are not from God. ☐

- Be determined to become slim and you will. Think differently, and it will be accomplished in the name of Jesus Christ! ☐

- Everyday, over the next seven weeks, read again the "Be determined…" list. ☐

NOTES

DEPROGRAMMING VIRUSES AND REPROGRAMMING ACCORDING TO THE WORD OF GOD

Applying the Principles

Done

- You have become a new creature in Jesus Christ. Think like a new creature of God. ☐

- Remove immediately all thoughts about your body and food which, are contrary to the will of God. ☐

- Diets and dietary restrictions are no longer part of your life. ☐

- Confess the truth of the Word of God over your body and in connection with your total deliverance from food. ☐

- You now see yourself as being free and slim. ☐

- You focus on what you want and not on what you do not want. ✳ ☐

- Do not look at the state of your body, but rather look at the state of your thoughts that will change your body. ✳ ☐

- Be proactive as soon as you wake up in the morning and glorify God for this miracle in your life. ☐

- Even if on some days you don't feel good about yourself, refuse and reject that emotion and that thought in the name of Jesus Christ, and repeat out loud that feel good in your body, you're slim and you're a marvelous creation. ☐

- Keep this book within reach everyday for the next seven weeks. Read and reread it. Your mind needs to be reprogrammed with the truth of God. ☐

- Stop nibbling out of habit, to pass the time, out of boredom, or to have something in your mouth. Eat only when you're hungry. ☐

NOTES

_____

_____

_____

_____

Understanding and Using Your Authority as a Child of God

Applying the Principles

Done

- Refuse the temptation of overeating (gluttony). ☐

- Be aware of the authority that was given to you and use it consistently at every moment! The Spirit that raised Jesus Christ from the dead lives in you. ☐

- Learn to release the five powers and command to your soul and your body to be free and slim. ☐

- Believe in God! Have faith! ☐

NOTES

THE POWER OF YOUR WORDS

Applying the Principles

I recommended you to repeat this sentence out loud, at least three times a day before eating:

"Thank you Lord for the marvelous creation that I am. My body is restoring itself like you originally created it. I eat and I stop when I'm full. I'm slim and beautiful and I'm at peace with food."

Done

- Make a list of all the negative words that were said about you and that you accepted and in turn, repeated to sabotage your self-esteem and destroy your body image. ☐

- Take authority over these words! Break them in the name of Jesus Christ and declare the truth according to the Word of God. ☐

- Stop and look at how you talk about yourself, your body, and food. Make it a habit of listening to your own words. Note the impact they have on your life. Enhance your self-esteem through biblical truths. ☐

Even if you don't believe it, by repeating the truth of the Word of God on yourself, you'll eventually believe it. The words of life and the power of God will then be manifested in your life. Your destiny will be filled with joy and freedom!

NOTES

_____

_____

_____

_____

_____

_____

_____

_____

_____

_____

_____

APPLYING THE
3 SPIRITUAL WEAPONS

Applying the Principles

Done

- Continue to practice all the keys and the teachings you received   since the beginning. ☐

- Every day of the week, say a prayer addressing your specific needs. ☐

- Fast with a goal that matches your needs and continue to use this weapon throughout the program. I suggest that you fast regularly during the coming weeks for 3 days per week during 7 weeks (a total of 21 days), or do a normal fast of 21 consecutive days. ☐

- Pray in tongues a few minutes per day, every day. Pray in the shower, in the car, while shaving or putting on make-up... ☐

- Ask the Lord for a specific amount to sow to get victory towards food and/or your body, where to plant that seed, and claim your harvest everyday. ☐

- Get a small notebook where you list all your seeds and keep your spiritual garden watered with prayers and the Word.

NOTES

6ᵀᴴ WEEK - DATE: _____

CRAVE FOR...

Applying the Principles

Done

- Ask God to live a passionate relationship with Him. ☐

- Make a list of the qualities that you like about yourself(personality, gifts, physical…). Stick this "for your eyes only" list is a place where you will see it frequently, such as your wardrobe. Read it each day, thanking the Lord for the wonderful creature you are. ☐

- Crave to be fulfilled. Find activities that you enjoy and be creative… ☐

- Move! Make one or more physical activities that you enjoy. ☐

- Cherish yourself through the choices you make towards food, exercises and the clothes you wear. ☐

- Consume good quality vitamins to compensate for deficiencies in the food you eat. ☐

- Sleep well. If you have trouble sleeping, this problem must be solved with the Lord's help.

- Surround yourself with people who are craving for you, what is inside you; people who raise you up, honor you and applaud your successes.

NOTES

_____

_____

_____

_____

_____

_____

_____

_____

_____

_____

PERSEVERENCE AND CONSISTENCY

Applying the Principles

Done

- Be perseverent and consistent in using your authority as a child of God. ☐

- Use perseverence and consistency in the way you talk about food and your body. ☐

- Persevere and be consistent in fasting (3 days x 7 weeks or 21 consecutive days), in sowing (the exact amount and place God puts in your heart) and in prayer. ☐

- You must persevere and be consistent in your craving for God, yourself, as well as surrounding yourself with people who crave for you. ☐

- And finally, be perseverent and consistent in applying this 777 Program day after day, week after week. ☐

- Repeat the 777 Program until you reach your goals. ☐

- Persevere to think as God thinks, and not as men do. ☐

- Persevere always. If some days are harder, if you fall... Pick yourself up and go on! ☐

- Remember that this key is as important as the other six. ☐

- You must be perseverent and consistent in your decision to be free and slim. ☐

- You must also be perseverent and consistent in the deprogramming of "viruses" and reprogramming according to the Word of God. ☐

NOTES

_____

_____

_____

_____

_____

_____

_____

Get now

the Be **Free**, Be **Slim**

Coaching CD!

The perfect complement to this book.

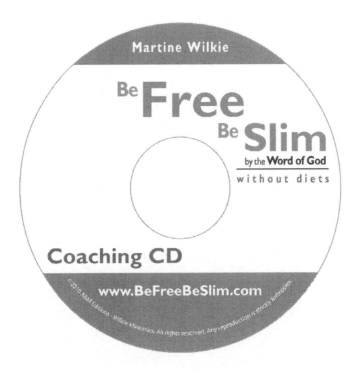

To order or to download right now:

www.BeFreeBeSlim.com

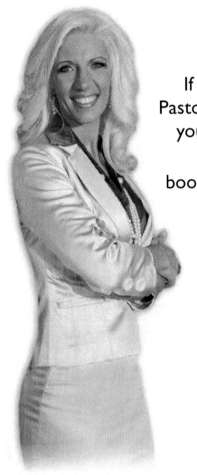

If you would like to have
Pastor Martine Wilkie speak at
your event, please contact:

booking@BeFreeBeSlim.com

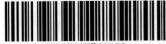

Made in the USA
San Bernardino, CA
13 April 2016